Women'sHealth
SHAPE-UP
SHORTCUTS

Shape-Up Shortcuts

CONTENTS

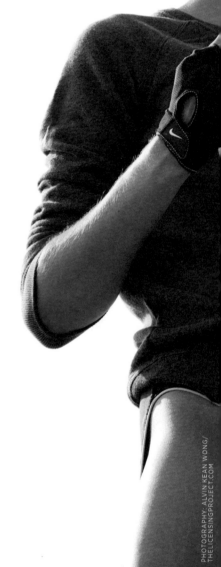

PHOTOGRAPHY: ALVIN KEAN WONG/ THELICENSINGPROJECT.COM

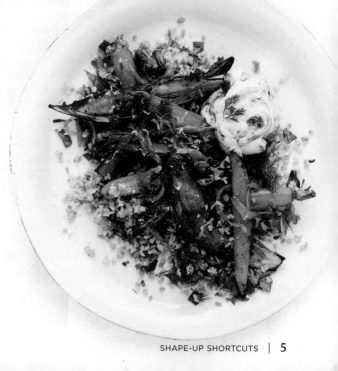

FOOD PHOTOGRAPHY: NATO WELTON.
FOOD STYLIST: NICOLE HERFT

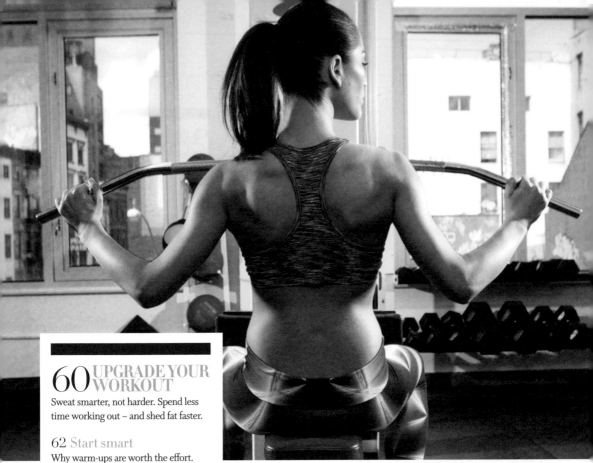

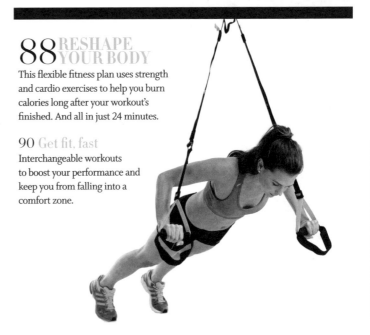

PHOTOGRAPHY: JUAN ALGARIN, NATHANIEL WELCH, WORKOUT PHOTOGRAPHY: BETH BISCHOFF

99 5-MINUTE FAT FIXES

Turbocharge your metabolism and make every one of those 300 seconds count.

100 Maximise every minute
If you're short on time, tired or can't make it to the gym, fear not. Five minutes is all you need to torch calories and sculpt muscle.

127 KEEP IT SIMPLE

Slim down faster, with less equipment.

128 The best-ever bodyweight workout
You don't need a gym membership – or even equipment – to sculpt a great body.

142 Tone every inch
Build a stronger, leaner body from head to toe with these three circuits.

148 One dumbbell, one hot body
Go fast and furious: incinerate fat and tighten your body in record time.

152 The ultimate kettlebell workout
How to burn up to 50% more calories.

158 Step up your results
Explosive, dynamic exercises build agility and speed – and burn calories.

162 The ball that does it all
Use a medicine ball to challenge your core stability and coordination, while toning your upper and lower body.

168 Sculpt a knockout body
Use a cable machine to sculpt your core and amp up your calorie burn.

173 CRUSH MORE CALORIES

Rethink your cardio routine, to boost endurance and keep burning calories.

174 7 Fat-blasting cardio workouts
Use these plateau busters to send your metabolism into hyperdrive.

176 Perfect your technique
Hit the great outdoors. Whether you're running, swimming or cycling, here's how to do it better and avoid injury.

180 Work out the kinks
Soothe aching muscles with this simple foam-roller routine. Soreness, begone.

185 STAYING ON TRACK

How to keep your focus and maintain your progress months down the line.

187 Four stages of burnout
Watch out for the warning signs, so you can sidestep that slump.

188 Outsmart fitness roadblocks
Distractions are inevitable – but these tips and tricks will keep you on track to a hotter, healthier body.

190 Stay motivated
Focus on immediate benefits – like feeling happier and more energetic.

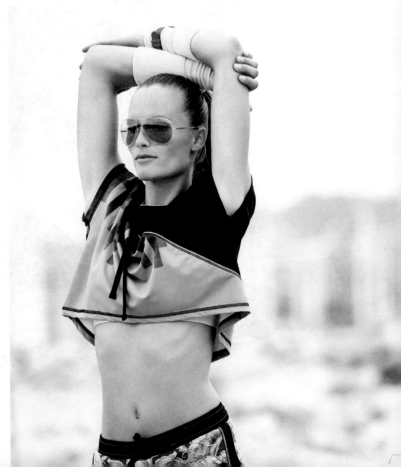

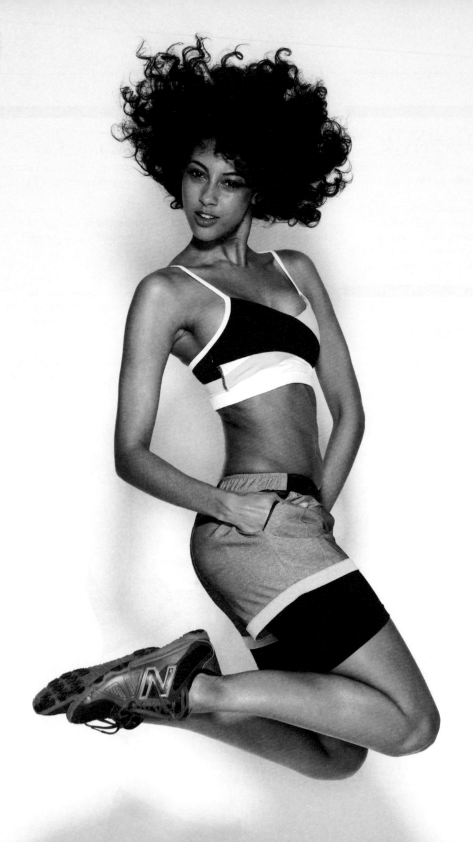

SMALL CHANGES
BIG
RESULTS

Here's your fast track to a leaner, healthier body

Some say there are no short cuts to any place worth going, but when it comes to achieving a hotter, fitter body, the direct route is easily the best. Done properly, it's actually quite easy to achieve lasting and healthy weight loss: by building sensible training habits and avoiding burn-out. Once you've nailed that and seen (and felt!) the changes, by all means, progress. Challenge yourself to longer, tougher workouts; hone your lean-eating. And don't worry if you fall off the wagon; this book will also help you climb back on. Either way, these short cuts are all about the thing that really makes the difference: simplicity.

WHY SHORTCUTS WORK

Keep your sweat-sessions short and sweet – it's the quickest route to fitness and good health

You'll get strong and stay that way

Just three 15-minute weight workouts each week can double a beginner's strength, say scientists at the University of Kansas. And unlike the average person, who quits her new exercise regime within a month, 96% of the study participants found they could easily fit shorter workouts into their lives, so they kept it up.

You'll blast belly fat

In an Australian study, women who cranked out high-intensity interval training three days a week for 20 minutes (for 15 weeks) shed more fat than those who exercised for 40 minutes at a lower intensity.

You'll make it manageable

Previously inactive women who exercised four times a week gained just as much fitness in 16 weeks as those who did six workouts a week. And they actually burned more total calories each day, reports a new study in the journal *Medicine & Science in Sports & Exercise*. How come? Those who exercised six times a week complained about not having enough time to get everything done, so they were more likely to drive instead of walk.

You'll push yourself hard (but not too hard)

If you think your workout is too tough, you're less likely to lose weight, reports the US journal *Obesity*. When women were asked to rate how hard a treadmill

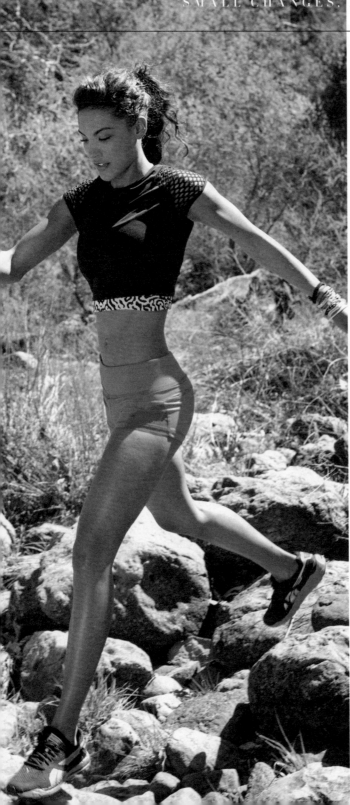

workout was, those who ranked it the toughest packed on the most pounds a year later. The study's authors found that when you have a negative experience with exercise, you're less likely to do it.

You'll keep torching calories

Just 10 minutes of moderate exercise dials up your metabolism for an hour or longer, reports the US journal *Science Translational Medicine*. Researchers found that levels of molecules involved in calorie burning changed significantly an hour after a 10-minute treadmill test, in some cases even doubling among the fittest participants.

You'll reduce your feelings of anxiety

Studies suggest that even small doses of regular exercise – about 10 to 20 minutes at a time – can improve mood and reduce anxiety. Exercise raises levels of serotonin, the feel-good chemical, while reducing your heart rate, blood pressure and stress hormone levels.

You'll build a stronger future

A little exercise goes a long way when it comes to protecting your bones and heart in later life. Research shows that just 10 minutes of high-impact exercise (like plyometrics) three times a week can boost women's bone strength – a critical factor in staving off osteoporosis as we age. And doing just 30 minutes of weight-training a week is linked to a 23% decrease in heart disease risk, according to Harvard researchers.

SIMPLE
SECRETS

... to getting a hotter body in half the time

Move a little, lose a lot

Most of us spend a terrifying 56 hours a week sitting, whether that's staring at a computer screen, behind a steering wheel, or collapsed in a heap in front of a high-definition TV. And when muscles (especially those in your lower body) are immobile, circulation slows and you burn fewer calories. Key flab-burning enzymes responsible for breaking down triglycerides (a type of fat) simply start switching off. Sit for a full day and those fat burners plummet by 50%.

And the less you move, the less blood sugar your body uses: research shows that for every two hours spent on your backside per day, your chance of contracting diabetes increases by 7%. Your risk of heart disease goes up too, because the enzymes that keep blood fats in check are inactive. Inactivity is also bad news for your posture and spine health. Your hip flexors and hamstrings shorten and tighten, while the muscles that support your spine become weak and stiff. And with less blood flow, fewer feel-good hormones are circulating to your brain, making you more vulnerable to depression.

Even if you exercise, you're not immune to these effects. We've become so sedentary that 30 minutes a day at the gym may not be sufficient to counteract the effects of eight, nine, or 10 hours of sitting. Many women still struggle with weight, blood sugar, and cholesterol woes, despite maintaining consistent workout routines. In fact, research shows that, regardless of how much moderate-to-vigorous exercise a person does, those who take more breaks from sitting throughout the day have slimmer waists, a lower body mass index and healthier fat and sugar levels in their blood than those who sit the most.

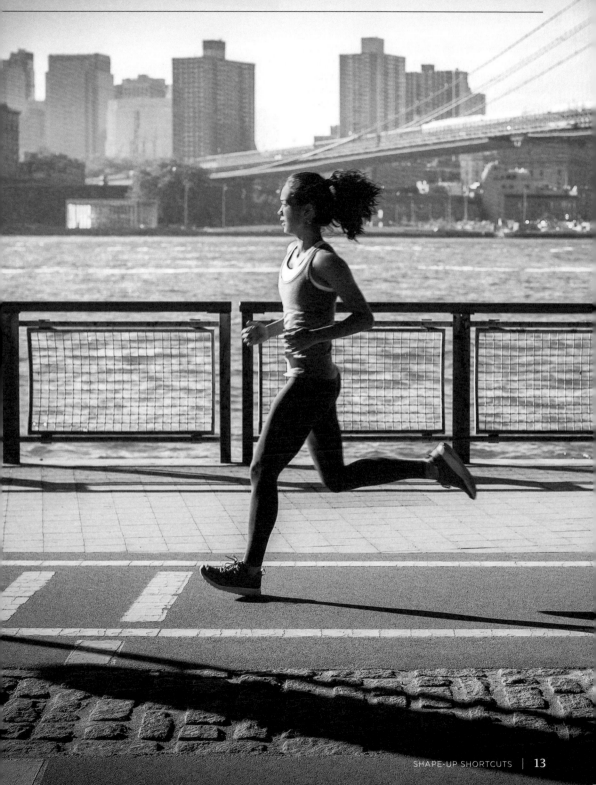

Recent research shows that getting into shape isn't an all-or-nothing proposition. In fact, you can make a significant impact on your waistline without ever setting foot in the gym. Folding laundry, tapping your toes, standing up on the bus, having sex, taking the stairs – all add up to make a vital difference. Research shows that lean participants move an average of 150 minutes more per day than overweight participants – enough to burn 350 calories. A University of Missouri study found that staying on your feet blasts up to 60 calories more per hour than sitting. Adding these simple activities can help stave off the 1-2lb weight gain that most women accumulate each year – and it can help to keep your metabolism fizzing in the way that nature intended. And getting up and moving around for roughly an extra hour a day has been shown to reduce stress and heighten your mood, energy, focus, and productivity.

Anything's better than nothing

Any amount of exercise is better than none, and research consistently proves that more frequent bursts of intense physical activity can produce the same muscle-building, fat-blasting, health-boosting benefits as the long-recommended 30 minutes a day. Studies have found that brief, vigorous workouts improve the body's ability to control blood sugar, and lower blood pressure more than longer, less-frequent sweat-sessions. Danish researchers found that participants who completed shorter workouts burned more calories than those who logged more drawn-out ones.

Even better, the results seem to be cumulative. A set of squats in the morning, a brisk walk at lunch, and some press-ups before bed will be just as beneficial as a marathon cardio session at the gym. And because a person can go all out for 60 seconds but not 60 minutes, mini-workouts can actually be more effective at sending your metabolism into overdrive, increasing your calorie-burn during and after each fitness blast.

Think 80:20 instead of all or nothing

Most of us can be disciplined for short periods, which might translate into a month of early-morning spin classes and salads with no dressing. The problem? Almost anyone can soldier through a brutal month of overtraining and calorie restriction, but research consistently shows that we can't keep it up for long periods of time. It's simply unsustainable – physically and mentally. So as soon as life gets in the way and there's a week when we can't get to the gym or down an entire tub of Ben & Jerry's after a hideous day or – all of a sudden the wheels come off. And it's

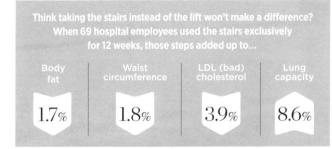

Think taking the stairs instead of the lift won't make a difference? When 69 hospital employees used the stairs exclusively for 12 weeks, those steps added up to...

Body fat	Waist circumference	LDL (bad) cholesterol	Lung capacity
1.7%	1.8%	3.9%	8.6%

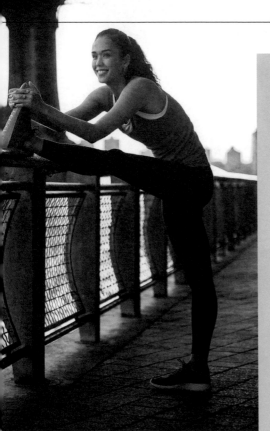

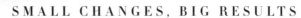

SET A GOAL

Goals are key – they're what keep you focused when the going gets tough. Use these six principles to make sure your goals are keeping you on the path to success

Be specific Vague goals give people too much flexibility. Set out to just 'tone up' and you're going nowhere. So be precise and say, for example, that you want to lower your body fat by 10%, or be able to run a 10K.

Make It Measurable You should be able to gauge and quantify your progress, both in the short and long term. Set weekly and monthly goals to keep yourself on track.

Stay Within Reach If you can barely find 20 free minutes in your day, don't set yourself up for failure by saying you'll run for 50 minutes three days a week.

Accept Reality Even with the smartest plan and the strongest determination, your body can only handle so much. Of course, fast weight loss is possible, but if you drop more than about a pound and a half a week, you're probably losing muscle and water – not fat.

Time it right Deadlines help maintain a sense of significance and keep your goals a priority.

Give yourself a year to drop 75 to 100lbs, four to six months to train for a marathon (if you're a new runner), and two months to lose 10-12% of your body fat.

that all-or-nothing approach that means one slip-up equals complete failure – so we give up.

This start-stop pattern usually leads to significant decreases of body weight (generally 10lbs or more), followed by equally significant increases – and it's usually not a one-time deal. According to a study published in the journal *American Psychologist*, dieters successfully lost up to 10% of their weight within the first six months on any number of diets. The problem is, nearly two-thirds of dieters put the weight back on (often gaining more) within five years.

This can change your physiology, increasing levels of the appetite hormone ghrelin and decreasing those of leptin, the hormone that is thought to make you feel full. And the more diets you've been on, the harder it becomes to lose weight. Researchers from Columbia University in New York found that dieting can slow your resting metabolism, so it's harder to maintain a stable weight post-diet. They reported that dieters may burn up to one-quarter fewer calories during exercise than those naturally at the same weight.

Your relationship with healthy eating and exercise doesn't have to blow hot and cold. Ignoring strict guidelines is often the secret to a successful slimdown. A study published in the *International Journal of Obesity* found that people with a flexible approach to eating – one that allows for slip-ups – had a better track record of maintaining weight loss than dieters with an all-or-nothing strategy. If some days you're too busy to exercise, or you end up eating pizza instead of steamed fish and broccoli, don't give up. It's the bigger picture that matters. And it's what you do most of the time that makes the difference. When overweight subjects in a study made several small lifestyle shifts, like eating a healthy breakfast, or having as many vegetables as they wanted with each meal, and watching TV for only as long as they'd exercised that day – they dropped an average of eight pounds in two weeks. And, more importantly, they managed to keep it off.

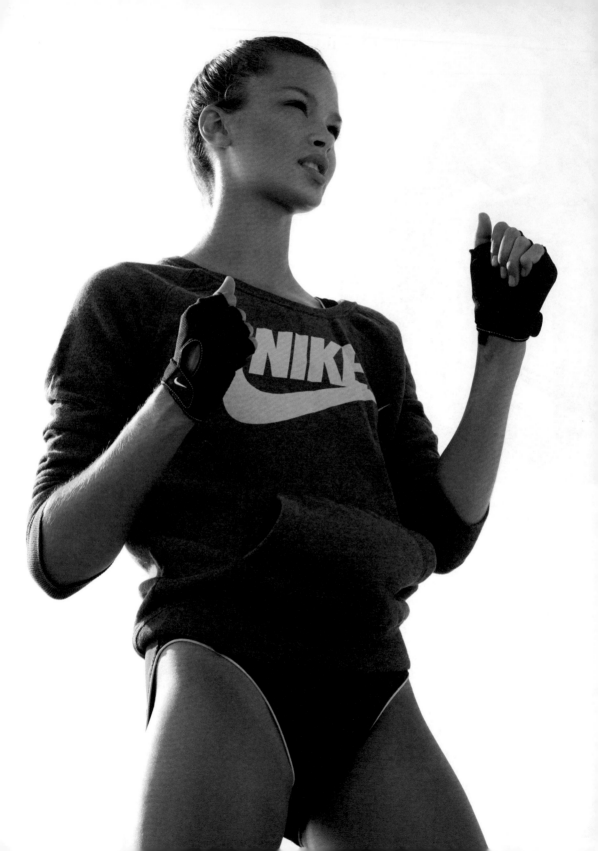

LOOK
HOT
IN A HURRY

Tackle any deadline – without losing the plot

Weight loss is a straightforward equation: calories in must be fewer than calories out. But to be truly effective, your time-crunched strategy must be tailored to your specific circumstances: the time you have until your big event; the number of pounds you need to lose; what kind of shape you're in. In any case, you must avoid the fitness and diet mistakes that can slow or derail your progress. Use the tips in this chapter to help you work out more effectively and pace yourself for fast, but not fleeting, results. However ambitious your goal or tight your time-frame, here's how to plan a trim-down timeline that will work for you.

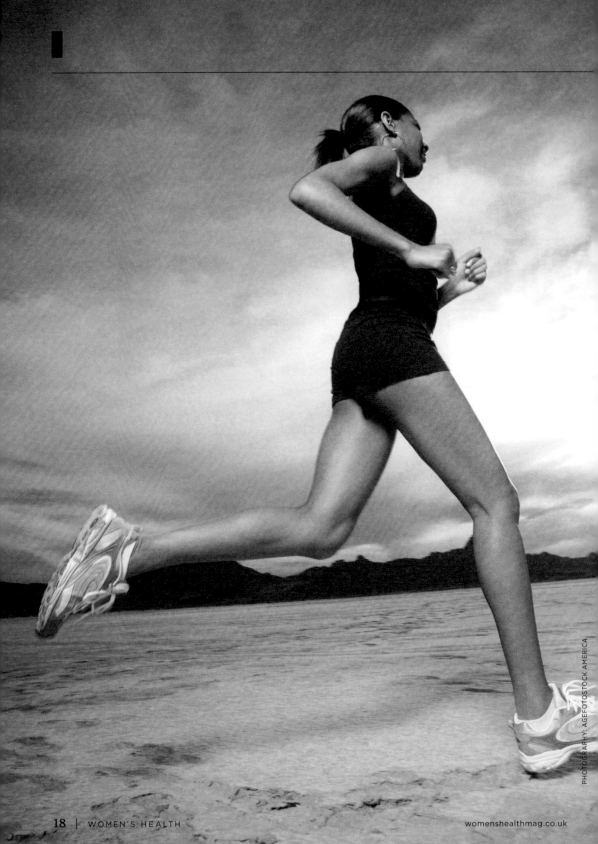

THE *FASTEST* WAY TO LOSE . . .

20lbs

Your goal weight may seem far off, but don't sweat it. The more you weigh, the more calories you burn during easier workouts, like brisk walking. Small, consistent efforts will help you shed pounds early on – and seeing those quick results will motivate you to stay on track.

Strength prescription: stay off the sideline
Your biggest challenge is keeping injuries at bay. Excess weight makes exercise naturally harder on your joints. Start with basic bodyweight exercises two days a week; they put less strain on your body and help you learn proper form. The Greatest Bodyweight Workout Ever on page 128 is built to adjust with you. Once you master the fundamental moves, your joints and muscles will be ready to tackle trickier exercises.

Cardio prescription: nice and easy
Slow and steady is the best approach, it's key to developing endurance, a crucial building block. Sustained, moderate-intensity cardio slowly introduces your joints to impact, reducing your injury risk. It also helps teach your body to utilise fat as fuel, so that you begin to burn more of it. Two days a week, aim to complete 30 to 45 minutes of cardio (you can walk, hike, bike, or swim). Mix up your routine to train different muscles and beat boredom. And pay attention to your body: it's better to do too little than too much.

10lbs

Breaking this double-digit barrier can be frustrating. Your body adapts to exercise over time, which can cause your metabolism to fall into a lull. Your body got fitter, and now your usual routine isn't enough.

Strength prescription: increase your weights
The secret to sailing into double digits is strength training three times a week – and not with 3lb dumbbells. Adding resistance helps you torch more calories during and after your workout, while replacing body fat with lean muscle mass. It's important to track your progress during workouts. When you hit a plateau, increase one of these four things: frequency (go from three workouts a week to four); intensity (if you've been using 10lb dumbbells, go to 15); time (increase your workout duration by five minutes); or type (if you've been doing the same routine, mix it up).

Cardio prescription: pick up the tempo
Now that your body is ready, dial up your cardio with tempos – longer intervals done at a moderately difficult intensity. The goal is sustained intensity, so you burn more calories in less time. You should be able to talk while you exercise, but not easily.

5lbs

The closer you get to your ideal weight, the tougher it is to reach it. Your body is always working to maintain its natural balance, so the more weight you lose, the harder your body works to hold on to it.

Strength prescription: turn up the energy
Plyometrics can shake your body out of its comfort zone. These explosive moves are great muscle builders, get your heart rate up and work multiple muscles simultaneously. They will strip that last layer of fat to show off the lean physique you've been building. Try doing as many burpees as you can in a minute, or the Step Up Your Results workout on page 158.

Cardio prescription: fast and furious
To kick your fat-burning into overdrive, make your cardio as explosive as your strength training. High-intensity interval training involves quick, sprint-like bursts, combined with periods of rest or easy recovery. Twice a week, complete an interval using the cardio of your choice. Then boost your weekly calorie burn with an extra day of cardio: 30 to 45 minutes at moderate intensity (or 65 to 80% of your maximum heart rate).

LOOK
YOUR BEST
IN...

Six weeks

Write out a manageable schedule you can stick to for at least five weeks. A study in *Health Psychology* reports that it takes new exercisers that long to make their sessions a habit. To prevent burnout, aim for consistent (four to five days a week), moderate workouts. Too many days off in between workouts can decrease drive, especially when your deadline feels so far away. Cap each session at 30 minutes, to make sure your muscles can recover. The Get Fit Fast workouts on page 90 are perfect: 24-minute sessions that check off strength training and cardio, three times per week.

Food for thought: Think replace rather than trim. Cutting calories too drastically this far out can feel too taxing. Instead, make one replacement each meal, to get more nutrients, like healthy fats, fibre, and protein into your diet. It's as simple as sprinkling toasted pumpkin seeds on your lunchtime salad, or adding a handful of fresh spinach to your pasta sauce at dinner.

Four weeks

The same basic rules apply at four weeks, especially if you're a beginner or it's been a few months since you've last worked out. In fact, people in these categories will probably struggle the most: managing their eagerness for results, while giving their body enough of a break-in period to adjust to the new routine before dialling up the intensity. Use the same Get Fit Fast workouts, but focus on two areas of your execution: load and tempo. You'll get the best results by choosing a weight that really challenges you to finish the set. At the same time, complete each rep as fast as possible, with good form.

Food for thought: Follow the 80-20 rule. About 80% of the foods you eat should be lean protein (such as poultry, fish and beans), fruits and vegetables, low-fat dairy, high-fibre grain products, and healthier fats such as olive oil. The other 20% can be foods that are not as healthy.

Two weeks

Motivation and dedication can work in your favour here. In this short window, it's easier to stay focused and committed. Plus, your body can tolerate a few extra sweat-sessions, if you train smart. Supercharge your metabolism by choosing any three strength workouts in this book and add two high-intensity intervals

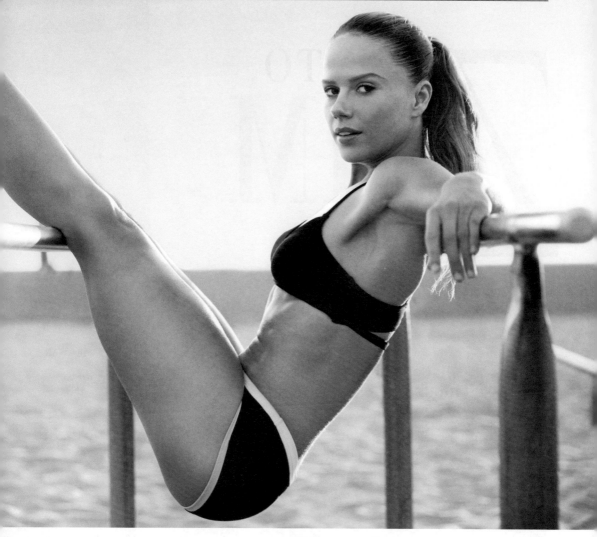

PHOTOGRAPHY: TURE LILLEGRAVEN

per week (find options in Crush More Calories on page 173). Whenever you increase the intensity, it's important to keep injuries at bay. Choose at least one low-impact cardio choice (such as swimming and cycling) each week.

Food for thought: Cut back on carbs. It's one of the most reliable strategies for short-term weight loss. Dutch researchers found that eating one carb-free meal a day over a two-week period can increase metabolic rate by 81 calories per day. The key is making the meal about 70% protein, and, of course, zero carbs. Watch for sneaky carb sources like milk and sausages.

One week

It may sound counter-intuitive, but scaling back your workout frequency and intensity could help keep you on track. Keep your routine light and manageable: walk 10,000 steps each day and complete one or two light strength-training workouts each week. While doing tons of cardio will undoubtedly burn extra calories, it could also ramp up your appetite.

Food for thought: There's no sense in starving. Eventually, inevitably, you'll end up breaking down and overeating. Follow the 7 Days To Slim plan (overleaf) to make smart and targeted changes.

7 DAYS TO SLIM

Implement one simple tweak each day – and keep it up until crunch time. You'll feel lighter and firmer in just one week

SUNDAY
Eliminate all processed foods

If you can't pronounce the ingredients, the food is off-limits. Or try to eat foods that have no label at all.

MONDAY
Lay off the sauce

Not only are alcoholic drinks dehydrating and high in calories, they also make resisting nibbles difficult. Studies prove women consume more calories after drinking.

LOOK BETTER TOMORROW!

Last-minute weekend plans? Don't expect miracles, but here's what celebrity trainer Valerie Waters advises her clients to do in a pinch

Get moving Torch calories and spike your metabolism with a 20-minute, fast-paced strength circuit, using light resistance (or just your body weight).

Cut it out Say no to sugar, alcohol, sodium, and refined carbs (such as white bread and pasta), and limit fibre intake to about 25g a day. All this causes your body to retain water, making you look (and feel) bloated.

Dine in This dinner combination revs up your metabolism and helps eliminate extra water weight. Prepare 4oz of low-fat fish (such as halibut, cod, or tilapia) drizzled with a tasty, low-fat spinach sauce (blend two large handfuls of spinach, 2 teaspoons olive oil, and lemon juice to taste in a blender until smooth). Serve with roasted, non-starchy vegetables, such as green beans, asparagus or aubergines.

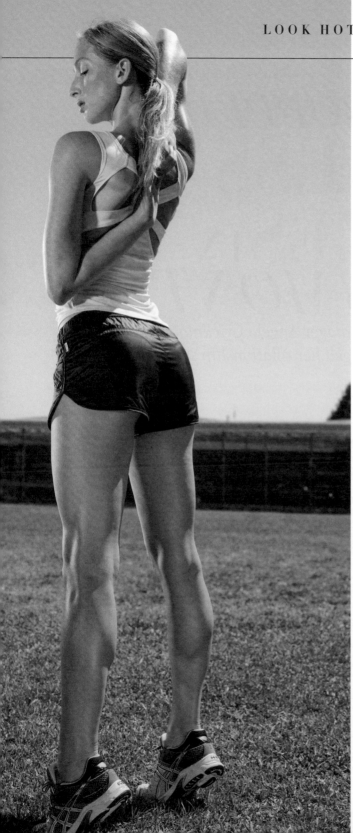

TUESDAY
Get a fibre fix
It may be tempting to forego all carbs, but don't forget fibre, a proven source of long-lasting satiety. Sprinkle flaxseed onto yoghurt, or add a few teaspoons of sliced almonds to your salad.

WEDNESDAY
Burn, baby, burn
Try to eat steadily throughout to day, it can prevent hunger (and snacking). Aim for three small meals (300 to 350 calories each) and two snacks (100 to 150 calories each).

THURSDAY
Banish bloat
Broccoli, cabbage, onions, and peppers cause bloating. Stick to apples, peas, cucumber, spinach and asparagus. Potassium-rich fruits, like bananas, avocados and oranges, also reduce self-induced bloating.

FRIDAY
Flush it out
Cells retain water when they don't have enough of it. Drink 2-3 litres each day. Sip slowly and the water will hit your bloodstream rather than filter out through your liver, so you won't have to pee every five minutes.

THE BIG DAY!
Befriend protein
A healthy, protein-rich breakfast will fill you up and head off unnecessary snacking. Think eggs!

'*I DROPPED* 6 DRESS SIZES IN *8 MONTHS*'

When accommodations manager Angela Crickmore, 35, changed her diet, she changed her relationship status, too

Then They call it 'relationship weight' – when you settle down and pile on the pounds. My ex-husband and I had rushed into marriage in 2003. As the years went by and cracks began to show, I was too unhappy to do anything about the comfort eating or creeping weight. Then, three years ago, I bumped into my beautician who'd been overweight for as long as I'd known her. But now she was svelte, glowing and happy. That was my lightbulb moment.

How I found studies online that said eating small portions every three hours was crucial to weight loss. I gave it a go. For breakfast, I'd have porridge and fruit; at 10.30am, a low-fat yoghurt and linseeds; for lunch, chicken with brown rice; at 4pm, a fruit salad or whey protein milkshake; three hours later, chicken with salad and vegetables. In the first week, I lost 4½lb. As my confidence grew, I started exercising – a few crunches at home at first, then I joined a gym, where I went five times a week. By now, my husband and I were eating separate meals. Our home life became incredibly tense and we split six months later.

Now It was a mutual decision, but I was devastated and terrified for the future. Yet, far from seeking solace in chocolate and ice cream, the gym became my way of coping. Now, two-and-a-half years on, I'm still at the gym five to six nights a week for 90 minutes at a time. I do 30 minutes' cardio, then weights. With each session, I work a different group of muscles: legs one night, abs, back and chest another. I'm not scared anymore. I'm enjoying my body and looking to the future.

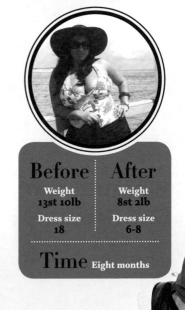

Before	After
Weight 13st 10lb	Weight 8st 2lb
Dress size 18	Dress size 6-8

Time Eight months

WRITER: CHRISTINA QUAINE. PHOTOGRAPHER: IAN HARRISON. ANGLEA WEARS: TOP, LEGGING; BOTH LUCAS HUGH; TRAINERS, NIKE. ANGELACRICKMORE.COM

'I USED TO BE A SIZE 18'

District nurse Gemma Butcher, 26, slimmed down and found the confidence to be in a relationship

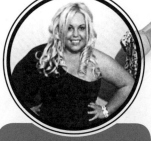

Before	After
Weight	**Weight**
14st 10lb	**8st 12lb**
Dress size	**Dress size**
18	**10**

Time 20 months

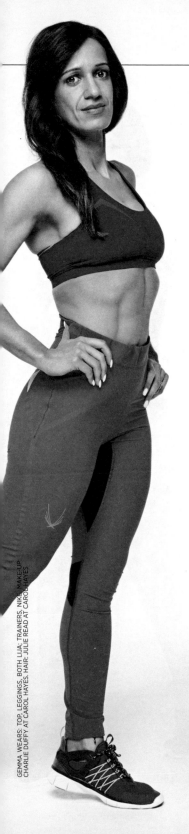

Then My early twenties were miserable. I'd been big since my teens, I'd skip breakfast, then would binge on junk. On nights I went out, I'd hide in the corner and I'd dread seeing the Facebook photos. In January 2012, another one popped up. There I was, unhappy in leggings and a loose-fitting top. Enough was enough.

How I adopted simple strategies, like eating breakfast and cutting back on sugar. I also joined a gym, which at first I hated. I did my own thing and stuck to cardio on the treadmill and StairMaster. Once I became a regular at the gym, I started recognising people – including a guy called Chris, but I was too shy to talk to him. It was May 2013, a year after I'd joined, when a friend I'd made there introduced us. We began dating and working out and suddenly I had extra motivation.

Now Eighteen months ago, I reached my target weight of 9st 8lb, but partly thanks to Chris introducing me to weightlifting, I managed to lose another 10lb – a weight I've stuck to. Saturday is treat night, but it's about making sensible choices – if Chris and I go for a curry, I pick dishes with lean meats and yoghurt-based sauces rather than rich, creamy ones. We're engaged and trying to set a date. I won't be slimming for the wedding – I've already got the man and the body.

'I LOST 4st IN 9 MONTHS'

PR manager Emma Stavrinides, 39, got in shape after she got a shock wake-up call from her GP

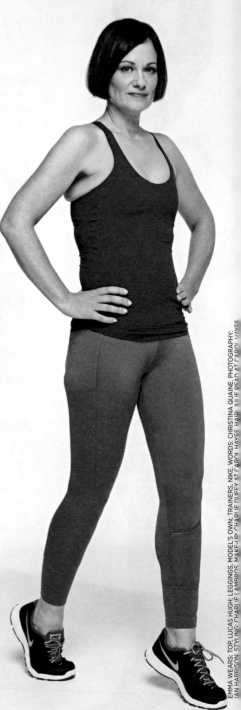

Then I was constantly run down, so my GP sent me for blood tests. The results were unexpected: I was borderline diabetic. It shouldn't have shocked me – I was an exhausted mum of two young boys and the weight had been creeping up since I'd given birth to my second son. I'd been diagnosed with postnatal depression and hadn't had the motivation to eat properly. I tried to tell myself my twice-weekly jogs were enough to keep me healthy, but at 15st, I knew I was lying to myself.

How I knew I had to cut the sugar out of my diet. I'd read about the blog Deliciously Ella and started following it. My dinners (creamy moussakas and cheesy jacket potatoes) were replaced with quinoa and roasted vegetables. For six weeks, I cut out refined sugar. The reality was agonisingly hard. I couldn't sleep, suffered headaches and was horrible to my husband Ari, but I stuck to it. I had grapes whenever I craved sugar. Within six weeks, my cravings were

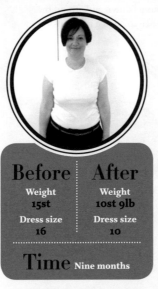

Before	After
Weight	**Weight**
15st	10st 9lb
Dress size	**Dress size**
16	10

Time Nine months

under control. I built my jogs up to six miles, three times a week and within just four months I was 2st lighter and on track to run a half-marathon.

Now When I returned to my doctor three months later, I was another 1st lighter – the nurse didn't recognise me. I was so happy when she told me my blood sugar levels were normal. I've since lost another 1st 5lb. It's just not feasible for me to live completely sugar free, so I follow the 80/20 rule, with good-quality chocolate or a glass of wine as treats. I'm still running three times a week and I do an Insanity class on Mondays. This summer, I'm celebrating my 40th birthday in Marbella. I'll be buying the brightest bikini I can find and wearing it with pride.

'I HALVED MY SIZE'

Insurance worker Alex Karaganis, 27, swapped secret binges for getting shredded at the gym

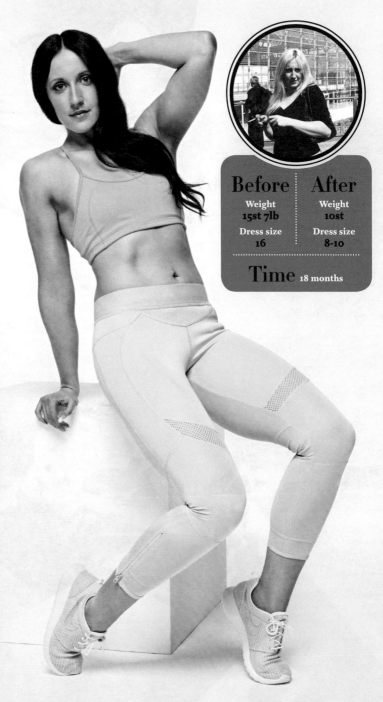

Then I'd always been overweight – singled out as the tubbiest girl in school. I felt embarrassed, under-ordering in restaurants and ashamed to let boyfriends see me naked. What people didn't know was that I'd binge in private. On my lowest days, I could get through three pizzas and 12 cans of pop. My weight caused constipation, high blood pressure, insomnia – I was constantly at my GP's. One day, in September 2011, he said that unless I changed, I faced obesity and heart problems. His words hit home.

How I signed up for a weekly Zumba class and soon built up to three classes a week. I knew my meals needed an overhaul. I realised I'd been consuming 3,000 calories a day! I set myself a healthy target of 1,200 calories and cut out all processed foods. Noticing my arms becoming toned and my fleshy belly more taut was more satisfying than a sugar fix. Six months later, I'd lost 3st and had the confidence to join a gym, where I took up weightlifting. I was hooked. It doesn't make you look bulky – I'm strong, not skinny.

Now Today, I don't recognise the overweight girl I used to be. I've gone from weighing more than 15st to training for a bodybuilding competition. I now dead-lift 140kg, eat 2,600 calories a day and have sculpted abs. I used to think being big was something I had to live with. But I'm proof that that's just not true.

Before	After
Weight 15st 7lb	Weight 10st
Dress size 16	Dress size 8-10

Time 18 months

ALEX WEARS: TOP, LIJA; LEGGINGS, MODEL'S OWN; TRAINERS, NIKE

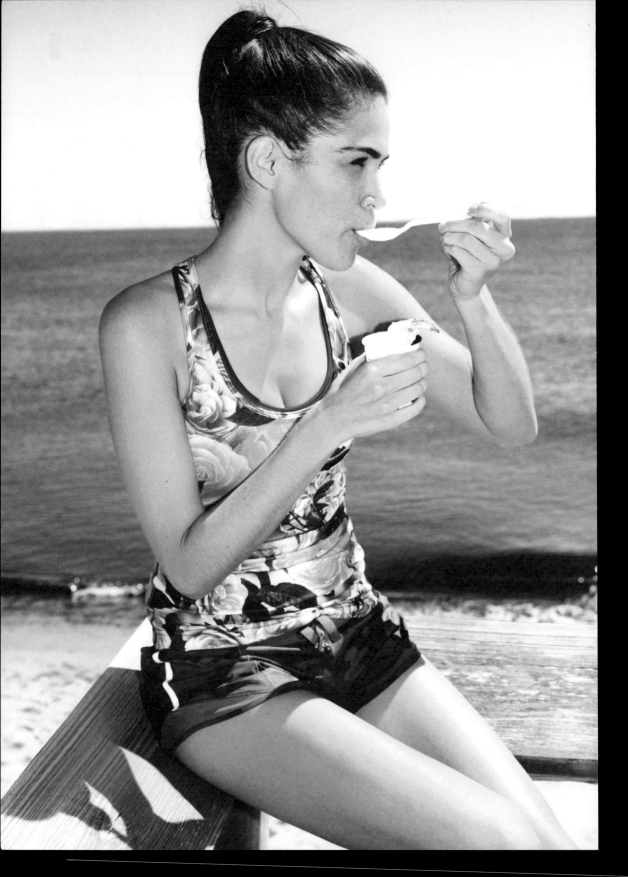

UPGRADE YOUR
DIET

...and reinvent your relationship with food

When your goal is fat loss, diet is one of the most – if not the single most – important pieces of the equation. Rather than strict diets that are impossible to maintain, eating well and enjoying the food you eat is the way to better health. And it doesn't have to be complicated: avoid processed foods and anything low-fat, and eat food in its most natural form. Cutting out refined sugar is the quickest way to look and feel better. If eating healthier rather than dieting means you cut just 96 calories from your daily diet, you'll be 10lbs lighter in a year – and that's before exercise or any strict diets. Even better, that weight will stay off.

SECRETS OF THE
SLIM

Learn to eat healthily, one meal at a time, by ditching deprivation and making small, significant changes

Take baby steps to better

Let's be realistic. You aren't going to swap crisps for kale chips, fried chicken for steamed fish, and ice cream for frozen berries overnight. Instead of going cold turkey, make the change from less healthy eats to better ones in baby steps. For the first week, don't even make it about the food, just focus on drinking six to eight glasses of water a day. Then, during the second week, trade half of your rice or pasta at dinner for the same amount of vegetables. Then ditch the top half of your bun from your burger, and so on. Rather than unbearable frustration followed by collapse, these small moves build confidence and teach your body to enjoy healthy foods that satisfy hunger.

Keep it consistent

Make sure your approach to eating is one you can stick with. Ask yourself, 'Can I see myself eating like this forever?' If the answer is no, you need to change your approach. Think of this as a permanent lifestyle shift. And consistency doesn't just mean Monday to Friday, either. Researchers have found that people who eat consistently day-to-day are one-and-a-half times more likely to maintain their weight loss than those who diet only on weekdays. But don't beat yourself up if you indulge occasionally. Follow up a fall from nutritional grace with healthy choices the next five times you eat. This means you'll be eating right more than 80% of the time. It's what you eat the majority of the time that most affects your waistline.

Take control

Planning a weekly menu and investing an hour or two on a Sunday will save you time and money, as well as pounds in the long run. Roast a chicken with some vegetables, then it's ready for packed lunches and weekday salads when you get home tired and hungry. Grill some marinated salmon and have it ready to go in the fridge – fish and salad is just as quick as pasta, but much healthier. Or buy a pack of smoked mackerel, add plenty of grated white cabbage, fennel and beetroot or carrot, top it with natural probiotic yoghurt and it's ready in less than ten minutes.

Planning your snacks helps, too. According to Dutch researchers, when asked 'What will you do if you get hungry two hours before your next meal?' thinner participants were more likely to, say, 'eat a handful of nuts'. And a survey by the US Centers for Disease Control and Prevention found that almost 40% of people who lost a significant amount of weight, and kept it off, planned their weekly meals. Otherwise, you're too tempted to eat high-calorie junk on impulse.

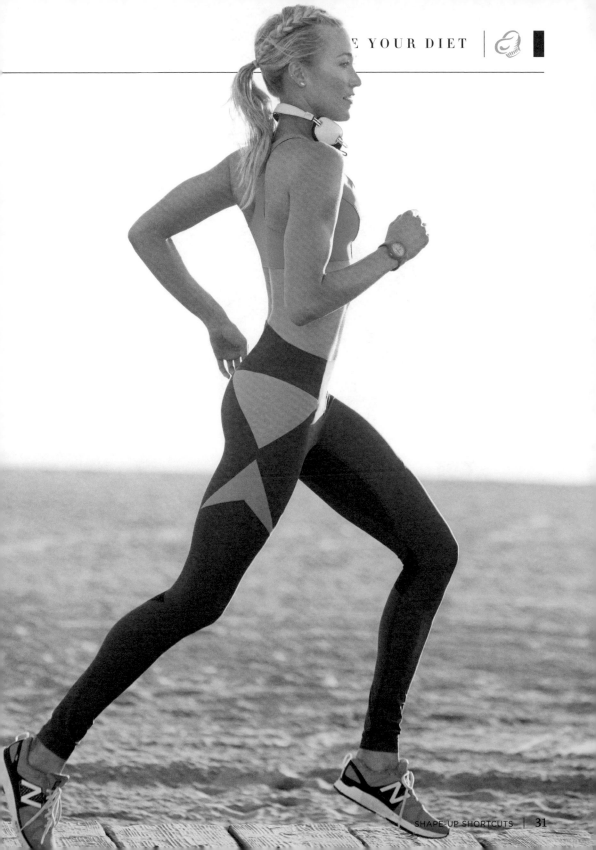

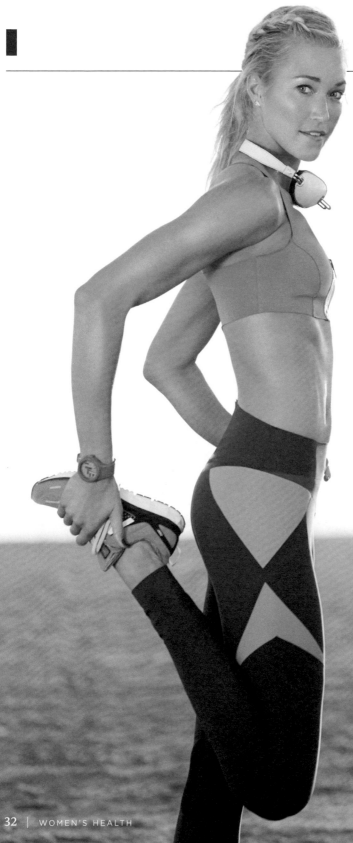

Find your own frequency

Forget eating three big meals a day. The 'graze, don't gorge' philosophy is based on the idea that having frequent small meals keeps your blood sugar steady, your metabolism up, and your appetite in check. Part of the logic is that going too long between meals (or skipping them) may lead to overeating later. It could even explain why women who skipped meals lost about 8lbs less than those who ate more consistently, according to a study in the US *Journal of the Academy of Nutrition and Dietetics*. But there's evidence that points the other way too. Other research shows a link between obesity and eating more than three times a day, most notably in women. After all, more frequent meals means more opportunities to overeat. The truth is, you'll eat healthiest if you eat your way. If you don't fancy breakfast, or if you prefer substantial meals fewer times a day, there's no reason to force yourself to eat when you're not hungry.

Keep it delicious

To be sustainable, you have to actually like, not just tolerate, the food you eat. But while a strict healthy eating regime can be a great tool for resetting your eating habits, if it's not tailored to your schedule, budget and personal preferences, it will fail. Of course if you cut out sugar, processed food or booze you'll shed some weight, but you probably won't keep it off. Start by making swaps that actually appeal, like chips for baked sweet potato wedges. You need to find healthier ways of feeling satisfied rather than deprived.

Size matters

According to researchers, our snacks have taken on meal-size proportions and our meals have become feasts. In one study, Pennsylvania State University researchers found that subjects ate 30% more food when presented with bigger portions, yet their perceived fullness didn't change. You could start your day with Greek yoghurt with fresh berries and granola,

DRINK AND STILL SHRINK
Dodge dieting pitfalls, even during happy hour

Between the drinks and the snacks, you can easily put away 1,000 calories before you've even thought about dinner. Alcohol stimulates your appetite and lowers your inhibitions, so the more you drink, the more likely you are to cave in to cravings. So, decide how many drinks you'll have before you embark on the evening's odyssey. And sip smart. Most wines and light beers have about 100-125 calories per serving. If you want something stronger, try a Manhattan (130 calories), mojito (150), or vodka tonic (170).

snack on an apple with peanut butter or carrots and houmous, eat a lunchtime salad topped with avocado, walnuts, hard-boiled eggs and feta cheese and end with brown rice, chicken, and roasted veggies for dinner. Fantastic, right? But even with the right kinds of foods, you can have too much of a good thing. Reduce your intake. We eat less from smaller plates and drink less from tall, narrow glasses.

Slow it down

Dutch researchers found that big bites and fast chewing can lead to overeating. Participants who chewed larger bites of food for three seconds consumed 52% more food before feeling full than those who chewed small bites for nine seconds. Tasting food for longer, even in small quantities, signals your brain to make you feel full sooner. But it can take up to 10 minutes for your brain to get the message that your stomach is full. The secret to avoiding this button-popping feeling of regret is to eat before you're completely starving (like, say, a six on a hunger scale of 10) and spend 20 to 30 minutes on a meal. This is long enough to get that satiety signal, but not so long that you'll be tempted to go for a second helping. And watch out during pudding. Levels of certain chemicals rise when people eat their favourite foods, reports the US *Journal of Clinical Endocrinology & Metabolism*, indicating that the food may turn on the brain's reward system, which overrides signals that you've had enough.

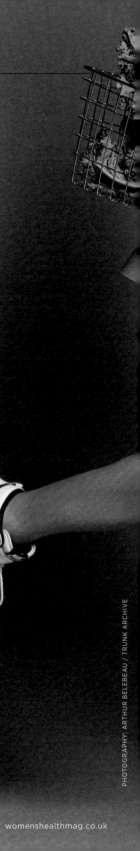

SUPERMARKET
SURVIVAL
GUIDE

The first step to eating delicious, fat-shedding meals is putting the right foods in your basket. These healthy eating tips will save you time, money and calories

DON'T BE A BASKET CASE

Dashing into the supermarket to pick up a few things? Don't grab a basket. If you're limited to what you can carry, you're more likely to avoid impulse purchases.

FLY SOLO

Your man may fancy fillet steak or your friend may tempt you with ice cream. Go shopping on your own and you'll be more likely to stick to the list you wrote before you left.

DON'T SKIP THE FREEZER AISLE

Because frozen and tinned produce are frozen or processed as soon as they're harvested, they're often more nutritious than fresh produce that's been shipped from all over the world. They're also more affordable and you can just take out what you need when you need it, so you waste less. Fresh, local produce

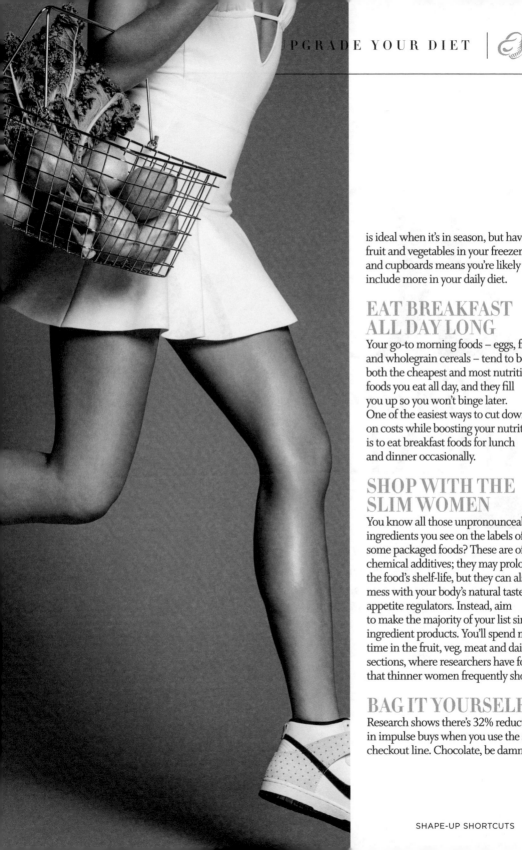

is ideal when it's in season, but having fruit and vegetables in your freezer and cupboards means you're likely to include more in your daily diet.

EAT BREAKFAST ALL DAY LONG

Your go-to morning foods – eggs, fruit and wholegrain cereals – tend to be both the cheapest and most nutritious foods you eat all day, and they fill you up so you won't binge later. One of the easiest ways to cut down on costs while boosting your nutrition is to eat breakfast foods for lunch and dinner occasionally.

SHOP WITH THE SLIM WOMEN

You know all those unpronounceable ingredients you see on the labels of some packaged foods? These are often chemical additives; they may prolong the food's shelf-life, but they can also mess with your body's natural taste and appetite regulators. Instead, aim to make the majority of your list single-ingredient products. You'll spend more time in the fruit, veg, meat and dairy sections, where researchers have found that thinner women frequently shop.

BAG IT YOURSELF

Research shows there's 32% reduction in impulse buys when you use the self-checkout line. Chocolate, be damned!

20 *Minute* MEALS

You can't out-exercise a bad diet, so put down that takeaway menu and get in shape with these speedy – and healthy – home-made dinners

📷

NATO WELTON

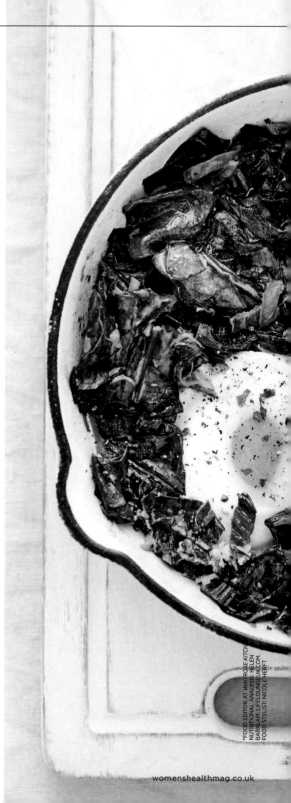

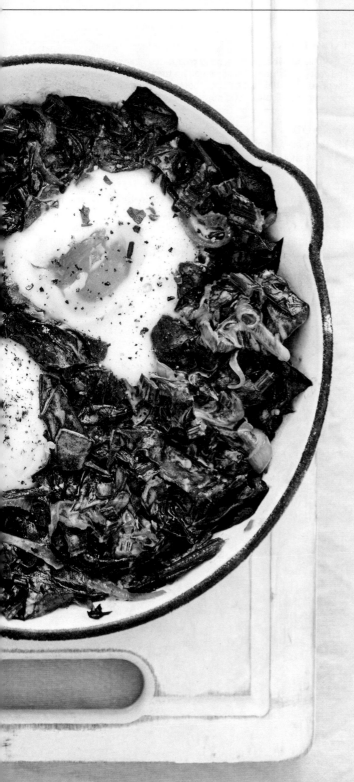

01

CHARD-BAKED EGGS

 SERVES 2 **CALS 377** **SAT FAT 6.4g** **SUGAR 4.7g**

INGREDIENTS
- 600g **chard** • 1 tbsp **olive oil** • 2 **banana shallots**, sliced • 4 **anchovies** in olive oil, drained • 2 **garlic cloves**, crushed
- pinch **chilli flakes** • 2 tbsp **single cream**
- 4 **eggs** • 1 tbsp chopped fresh **dill**
- dash **Tabasco sauce**

METHOD
1 Separate the chard leaves and stalks. Finely chop the stalks and sauté in a large frying pan with the oil and shallots for 5 mins. Finely chop the anchovies and add to the pan with the garlic and chilli flakes for another 2 mins. Toss in the roughly chopped chard leaves, cook for another couple of minutes until wilted, then stir in the cream and season with black pepper.
2 Turn the heat to low. Using a spoon, make four holes in the chard mixture and crack in the eggs. Cover the pan with a lid (a large plate or sheet of foil will work) and cook for 5 mins until the eggs are set. Scatter over the dill and add a dash of Tabasco. Brunch, reinvented.

02

SUMAC TUNA TABBOULEH

SERVES **4** · CALS **335** · SAT FAT **1.1g** · SUGAR **3.4g**

INGREDIENTS

· 150g **bulgur wheat** · 200g **baby courgettes** · 2 tbsp **olive oil** · juice and zest of ½ **lemon** · 2 tbsp **sumac** · 4 **tuna steaks** · 6 **spring onions**, chopped · 50g **flat-leaf parsley**, chopped · 25g **mint leaves**, chopped · pinch ground **allspice** · 50g **pomegranate seeds**

METHOD

1 Soak the bulgur wheat in a large bowl with enough boiling water to cover. Leave for 20 mins.
2 Cut the courgettes lengthways and toss with 1 tbsp oil and the lemon zest. Cook on a searingly hot griddle, cut-side down, for 4 mins, then flip and cook for 2 mins.

3 Mix the sumac and remaining oil and brush over the tuna steaks. Cook on the hot griddle for 1-2 mins each side. Fluff the bulgur with a fork and toss with the courgette, spring onions, herbs, lemon juice, allspice and pomegranate seeds. Pile onto plates with the tuna. Now, dig in.

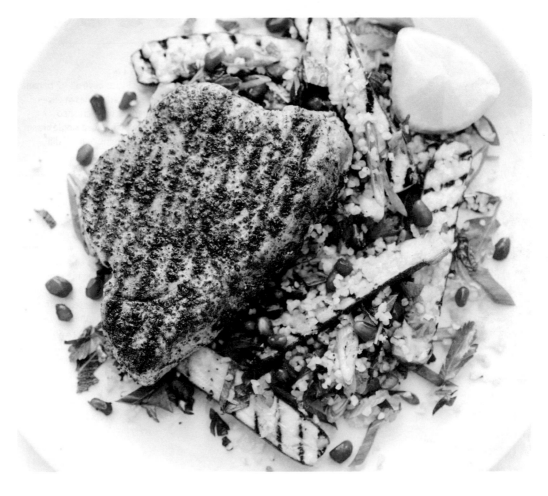

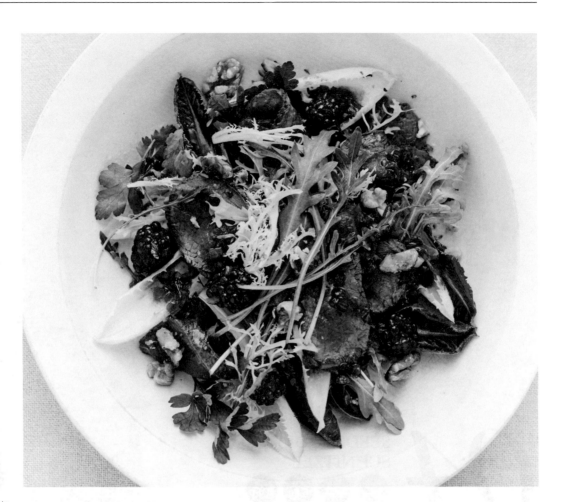

PHOTOGRAPHY: NATO WELTON, FOOD STYLIST NICOLE HERFT

03

WARM VENISON AND BLACKBERRY SALAD

SERVES
4

CALS
342

SAT FAT
1.25g

SUGAR
6.08g

INGREDIENTS

• 3 **venison steaks** (150g each) • 1 tbsp **olive oil** • 2 tbsp **walnut oil** • 1 **shallot**, finely diced • 3 **juniper berries**, crushed • 1 **thyme sprig** • 100g **blackberries** • 1 tbsp **sherry vinegar** • 1 tsp **honey** • 4 heads **white and red chicory**, leaves roughly chopped • 50g **curly endive** • 10g **flat-leaf parsley** • 100g **wild rocket** • 50g toasted **walnuts**

METHOD

1 A hearty salad, this one. Heat a frying pan on high heat. Rub the steaks with olive oil, season and cook for 3 mins each side. Set aside to rest under a sheet of foil.
2 Return the pan to low heat, add the walnut oil, shallot, juniper and thyme and sauté for 5 mins until soft, scraping up any caramelised bits from the pan. Add the blackberries, then stir in the vinegar and honey.
3 Slice the venison and place in a bowl with the walnuts, chicory, endive and rocket. Toss with the dressing and a grind of salt and pepper. Serve immediately.

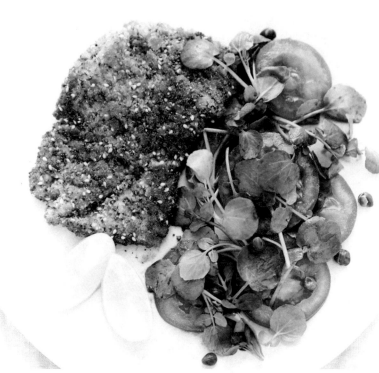

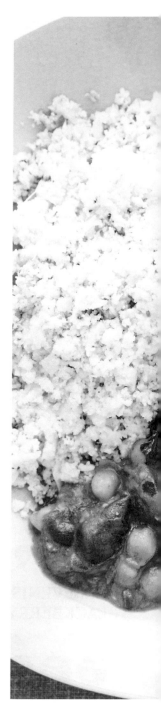

04

SEEDED PORK SCHNITZEL

SERVES	CALS	SAT FAT	SUGAR
4	600	6.8g	5.9g

INGREDIENTS
3 tbsp **plain flour** •
2 **eggs**, lightly beaten •
75g **breadcrumbs** • 75g
sesame seeds • 2 tbsp
flaxseeds • 2 tbsp **chia
seeds** • 4 **pork escalopes**
(120g each) • 100ml
vegetable oil • 1 tbsp
English mustard • 1 tbsp
olive oil • 1 tbsp **balsamic
vinegar** • 500g **tomatoes,
sliced** • 1 tbsp **capers** •
100g **watercress** • 1 **lemon**

METHOD
1 Grab your apron, things could get a bit messy. Put the
flour in a shallow dish; beat the egg in another; mix the
crumbs and seeds in a third, with plenty of seasoning.
2 Season the escalopes and, one by one, dust with
the flour; then dip in the egg; then coat well in the
seeds. Heat the oil in a large frying pan and fry over
medium heat for 4-5 mins on each side.
3 Meanwhile, whisk the mustard, olive oil and balsamic
together. Toss with tomatoes, capers and watercress
and season. Drain the schnitzel on kitchen paper and
serve with salad and lemon wedges. Dig in.

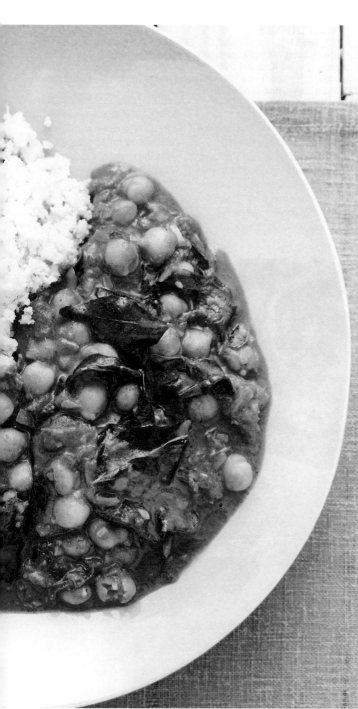

05

CHICKPEA CHILLI CURRY

SERVES	CALS	SAT FAT	SUGAR
4	434	11.5g	4.6g

INGREDIENTS

2 tbsp **ghee** · 2 **shallots**, chopped · 2 **garlic cloves**, crushed · 20g **ginger**, grated · 1 **green chilli**, chopped and deseeded · handful **curry leaves** · **cinnamon stick** · 1 tsp **curry powder** · ½ tsp **ground turmeric** · 227g tin **chopped tomatoes** · 400ml **coconut milk** · 2 x 400g tins **chickpeas** · 1 **cauliflower** · handful **baby spinach**

METHOD

1 Put down that takeaway menu and heat the ghee in a large pan instead. Gently sauté the shallots, garlic and ginger for 2-3 mins. Add the chilli, curry leaves, cinnamon and spices and cook for another 2 mins. Tip in the tomatoes, coconut milk, chickpeas and a pinch of salt. Bring to the boil, then turn down to simmer for 10 mins, adding a splash of water if it looks like it might be drying up. **2** For the cauliflower rice, first trim and discard the outer leaves and stem. Roughly chop the cauliflower into chunks and pulse in a food processor until it resembles rice. You can serve it as is, or dry toast it in a frying pan for a few minutes. Stir the spinach into the curry until the leaves have wilted, then serve with the cauliflower rice. Mango chutney: optional. Excitement: compulsory.

06

TANDOORI LAMB SKEWERS

SERVES	CALS	SAT FAT	SUGAR
4	524	28.3g	1.9g

INGREDIENTS

400g **lamb leg**, in 3cm chunks • 2 tbsp **tandoori paste** • 1 tbsp **lemon juice and zest** • 1 tbsp **coconut oil** • 1 **garlic clove**, sliced • 1 tsp **cumin seeds** • 1 dried **Kashmiri chilli** • 150g **baby spinach** • 450g **coconut milk yoghurt** (try Coyo) • handful **coriander leaves** • pinch **cayenne pepper** • 250g **brown rice**, cooked

METHOD

1 Toss the lamb with the tandoori paste, lemon juice and zest. Thread onto 8 skewers and leave to marinate for a good long while. **2** Heat up the griddle pan, then sear the skewers on it for 8-10 mins until cooked and nicely charred; set aside to rest.

3 Heat the coconut oil in a frying pan, add the garlic, cumin and chilli and fry for 30 seconds, then tip in the spinach and toss until wilted. Stir through the yoghurt and scatter with coriander and cayenne. Serve with the lamb and brown rice. Any leftover lamb will make great sandwiches.

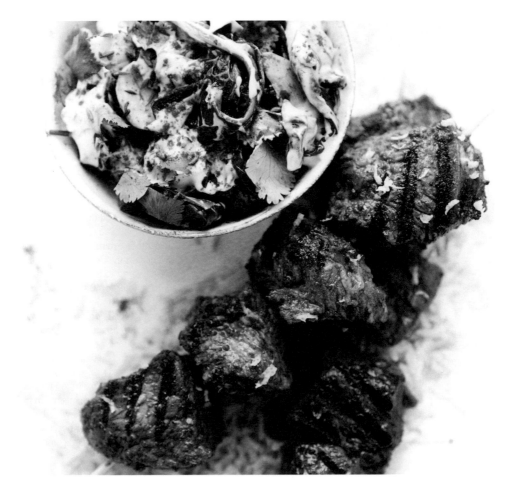

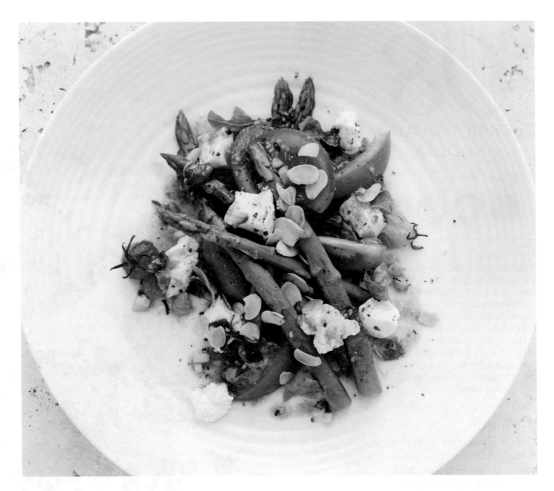

07

ASPARAGUS TOMATO SALAD

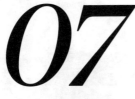

 SERVES **4**

 CALS **269**

 SAT FAT **3.1g**

 SUGAR **5g**

INGREDIENTS

150g **cherry tomatoes** • 2 **garlic cloves**, skins on • 2 **thyme sprigs** • 4 tbsp **extra-virgin olive oil** • ¼ **lemon** • 400g **asparagus** • 3 **tomatoes**, in wedges • 150g **soft goats' cheese** • 2 tbsp **sherry vinegar** • handful **basil leaves** • handful **oregano leaves** • handful **toasted flaked almonds**

METHOD

1 Get your oven hot: 220°C hot. Toss the cherry tomatoes, garlic cloves, thyme and oil. Slice the lemon and scatter everything on a roasting tray. Cook for 18 mins, until the tomatoes blister and the lemon caramelises.
2 Simmer the asparagus for 2-3 mins in a pan of boiling water.

Drain, then spread over a platter with the larger wedges of tomato. Add blobs of the goats' cheese.
3 Take the tomatoes out of the oven, squeeze out the roasted garlic, mix in the vinegar and mash it all with a fork. Pour over the asparagus and scatter the herbs and almonds. Veggie bliss.

08
CRAB AVOCADO NOODLES

SERVES **4** · CALS **267** · SAT FAT **4.2g** · SUGAR **4.9g**

INGREDIENTS

2 **cucumbers** · 5 **spring onions**, sliced ·
2 **avocados**, roughly chopped · 1 **red chilli**,
finely sliced · 100g **radishes**, finely sliced ·
½ **Granny Smith apple**, finely sliced ·
10g **coriander leaves** · 200g fresh **white
crab meat** · ½ tbsp **toasted sesame
seeds** · ½ tbsp **black sesame seeds** ·
DRESSING 2 tsp **wasabi paste**
· 1 tbsp **mayonnaise** · 2 tbsp **low-fat
crème fraîche** · juice and zest ½ **lime**
· 1 tsp **runny honey**

METHOD

1 Time to whip out the spiralizer. Halve
the cucumbers, then spiralize to create
noodles (or use a vegetable peeler
to create long ribbons, discarding the
seeds). Toss the noodles with a pinch
of salt and leave in a sieve while you
prepare the rest of the vegetables.
2 For the dressing, stir the wasabi, mayo,
crème fraîche, lime juice, zest and honey.
3 Time to serve up. Place the cucumber
noodles in a large bowl with the spring
onions, avocado, chilli, radish, apple
and half the coriander and crab. Toss
with the dressing, adding more lime juice
and salt to taste. Pile onto a large platter,
top with the remaining coriander and
crab and scatter over the sesame seeds.

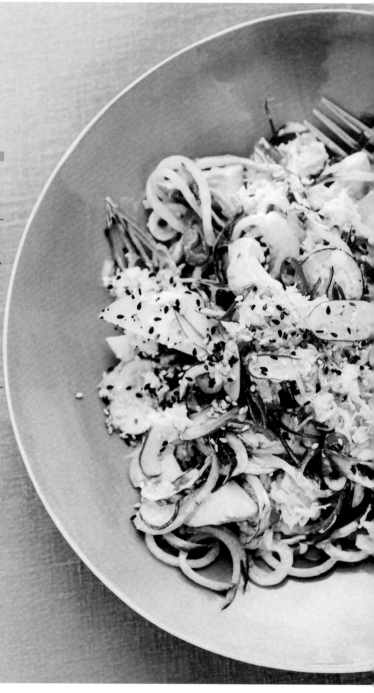

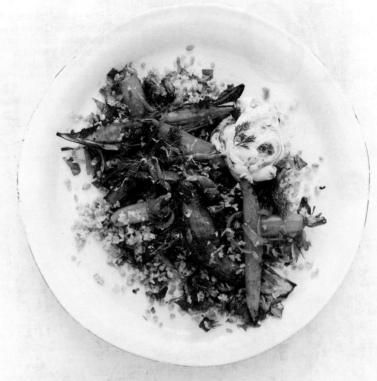

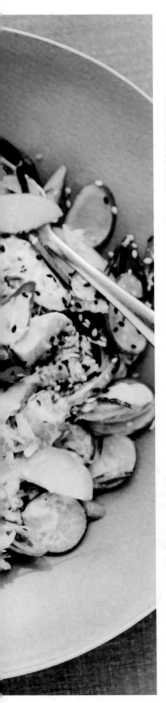

09

HARISSA FREEKEH

 SERVES 4 **CALS** 413 **SAT FAT** 4.3g **SUGAR** 7.7g

INGREDIENTS

½ tbsp **honey** • 2 **garlic cloves**, crushed • 2½ tbsp **harissa** • 2 **aubergines**, in wedges • 300g **baby carrots** • 2 tbsp **oil** or 1 tbsp **ghee** • 2 **onions**, sliced • ½ tsp ground **cinnamon** • ½ tsp ground **cumin** • 250g cooked **freekeh** • juice and zest of 1 **lemon** • 10g **dill**, chopped • 10g **mint leaves**, chopped • 2 tbsp **natural yoghurt**

METHOD

1 You like spicy? Heat the oven to 220°C. Mix the honey, garlic and 2 tbsp harissa and toss in a bowl with the aubergines and carrots. Season and spread out on a parchment-lined baking tray, and roast for 20 mins.

2 Meanwhile, heat the oil or ghee in a large frying pan and fry the onions for 10 mins. Add the spices and cook for 1 min, then stir in the freekeh, tossing everything together with the lemon zest, juice and herbs.

3 Spread the freekeh over a large platter, top with the roasted vegetables. Swirl the remaining harissa through the yoghurt and spoon over. Serve to glorious applause.

10

NAKED PORK BURGERS

 SERVES
4

 CALS
318

 SAT FAT
9.2g

 SUGAR
3.9g

INGREDIENTS

500g lean **pork mince** • 1 **small onion**, grated • zest ½ **lemon** • pinch **ground allspice** • ½ tsp **fennel seeds**, toasted and crushed • 1 tsp **olive oil** • 100g cooked **beetroot**, finely chopped • ½ **apple**, cored and finely chopped • 1 tbsp **creamed horseradish** • 1 tbsp **sour cream** • 1 tbsp chopped **dill** • 4 large **lettuce leaves**

METHOD

1 Sleeves up, it's time to get properly stuck in. Using your hands, mix the pork mince with the onion, lemon zest, allspice and fennel seeds. Season and fry off a bit of the mixture to check the seasoning, and when you're happy, shape into 4 burgers.

2 Get a griddle pan flaming hot, brush the burgers with the oil and cook for 6-7 mins on each side.
3 Squeal, piggy. While they're sizzling, mix the beetroot, apple, horseradish, sour cream and dill. Let the burgers rest, then wrap in lettuce leaves, piling on the relish. You won't even miss the bun.

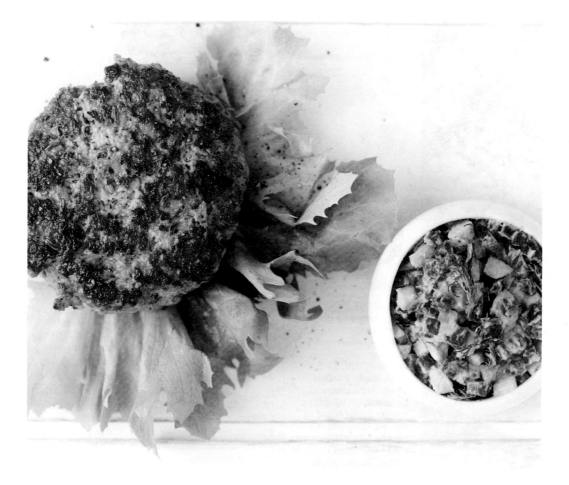

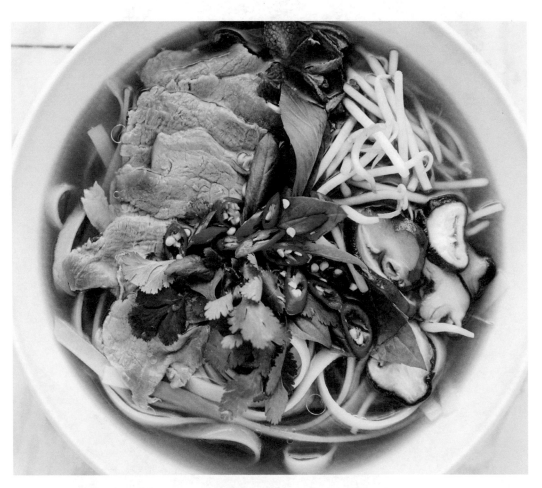

11

SHIITAKE & BEEF PHO

SERVES	CALS	SAT FAT	SUGAR
4	417	4.2g	2.5g

INGREDIENTS

1.5 ltrs **organic beef** or **chicken stock** • 3 **star anise** • 3 **cloves** • 1 tsp **fennel seeds** • 2 **lemongrass stalks** • 30g **fresh root ginger**, sliced • 1 **onion**, sliced • 2 tbsp **fish sauce** • 150g **shiitake mushrooms**, sliced • 300g **steak** (rump or sirloin) • 200g cooked **flat rice noodles** • handful **bean sprouts** • handful **Thai basil**, **mint** and **coriander** • 1 **red chilli**, sliced • 1 **lime**, in wedges

METHOD

1 Place the stock in a large pan with the spices, lemongrass, ginger and onion. Bring to the boil, simmer for 15 mins, then strain the liquid into a pan. Bring it back to a simmer, add the fish sauce and shiitake mushrooms and simmer for another 2 mins.

2 Finely slice the beef, add the meat to the stock and take it off the heat – it'll still cook.
3 Divide the rice noodles between 4 bowls. Ladle the stock over the noodles and top with the beansprouts, herbs, chilli and lime. Looking good? Pho shizzle. (Yes, we went there.)

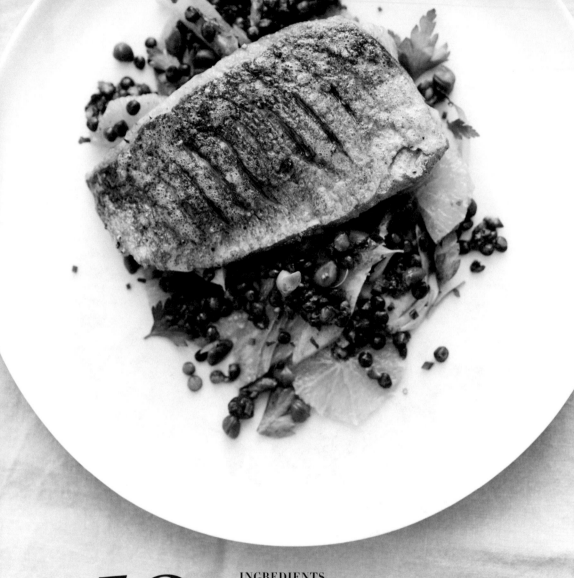

12

SEARED SEA BASS WITH FENNEL

 SERVES 4   **CALS** 382   **SAT FAT** 5.3g   **SUGAR** 6.6g

INGREDIENTS

4 **sea bass fillets** · 2 **fennel**, sliced · 30g **butter** · 1 **onion**, sliced · 200g cooked **lentils** · 150ml **stock** · 1 tbsp **capers**, rinsed · 1 tbsp **olive oil** · 1 **orange** · 1 tbsp chopped **chives** · 1 tbsp chopped **flat-leaf parsley** · 1 tbsp shredded **basil leaves**

METHOD

1 Heat 15g butter in a large frying pan. Sauté the fennel and onion for 6-8 mins until soft. Add the lentils, stock and simmer for 3-4 mins until most of the liquid has evaporated. Stir through the capers and remaining butter; set aside.
2 Meanwhile, rub the oil over the skin of the sea bass and season.

Fry skin-side down for 3 mins, then flip over and take off the heat. Leave for 3 mins to finish cooking.
3 Top and tail the orange, remove the skin and pith. Slice the flesh into rounds and toss through the lentils with the herbs. Pile onto plates and top with the sea bass. You know, it's all about that bass.

13

TARRAGON CHICKEN BROTH

SERVES **4** · CALS **269** · SAT FAT **3g** · SUGAR **5g**

INGREDIENTS

1 litre **fresh chicken stock** · 4 **tarragon sprigs** · 2 large **chicken breasts** · 4 each **baby leeks** and **baby carrots**, halved lengthways · 2 **baby fennel**, sliced · 200g **Jersey Royal potatoes**, sliced · 100g fine **asparagus** tips · 3 tbsp **half-fat crème fraîche** · juice and zest ½ **lemon**

METHOD

1 Bring the stock and 2 tarragon sprigs to a simmer in a shallow pan. Slip in the chicken, leeks, carrots, fennel and potatoes, simmer 8 mins, turning chicken halfway. **2** Add the asparagus and simmer 2 mins. Discard the cooked tarragon and stir through the remaining tarragon with crème fraîche, lemon juice and zest. Check the meat is cooked through, remove from pan and slice. Ladle into bowls, topped with the chicken. Voilà!

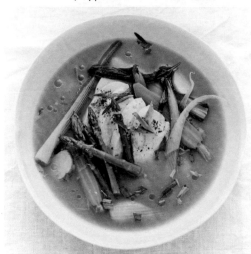

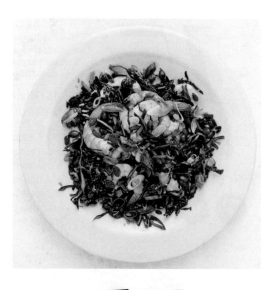

14

PRAWN & BLACK RICE

SERVES **4** · CALS **276** · SAT FAT **7.4g** · SUGAR **7.4g**

INGREDIENTS

100g **cavolo nero** · 100g **red cabbage** · 200g **black rice**, cooked · 300g cooked **prawns** · 6 **spring onions**, chopped · handful each **chives** and **mint**, chopped · 50g **rocket leaves** · 100g **pomegranate seeds** · handful **pumpkin seeds**

DRESSING 2 tsp **maple syrup** · 2 tbsp **balsamic vinegar** · 2 tbsp **rapeseed oil** · juice and zest ½ **orange**

METHOD

1 Preparation is key here – have everything ready. For the cavolo nero and cabbage, cut out and discard stalks and shred finely. **2** Mix all the dressing ingredients in a large bowl and season. Tip in the rice, then toss in the remaining ingredients. Serve piled up on a pretty platter – and marvel at your delicious and nutritious creation.

15

ROASTED CAULIFLOWER

SERVES 4 · **CALS** 142 · **SAT FAT** 7.5g · **SUGAR** 3.6g

INGREDIENTS

1 **cauliflower**, outer leaves discarded · 1 tbsp **coconut oil** · pinch **turmeric** · pinch **ground cumin** · pinch **ground cinnamon** · **pinch cayenne pepper** · 2 tbsp **tahini** · 2 tbsp **Greek yoghurt** · 1 tbsp **lemon juice** · handful **flat-leaf parsley leaves**

METHOD

1 This one's so ridiculously easy. Ready? Preheat your oven to 220°C. Boil a large saucepan of salted water, add the cauliflower and simmer gently for 8 mins.
2 Mix the coconut oil and spices, season well and set aside. In a separate bowl, mix the tahini, yoghurt and lemon juice with 3-4 tbsp water until it's the consistency of double cream. Mix in the herbs.
3 Drain the cauliflower and pat it dry with kitchen towel. Then place floret-side up on a foil-lined baking tray and rub in the spiced coconut oil. Roast for 10 mins. Let it cool, before tearing off the florets and dunking them in the tahini sauce. Ottolenghi, eat your heart out!

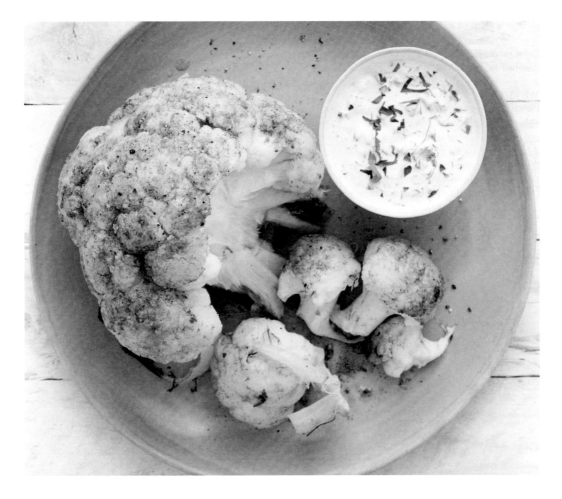

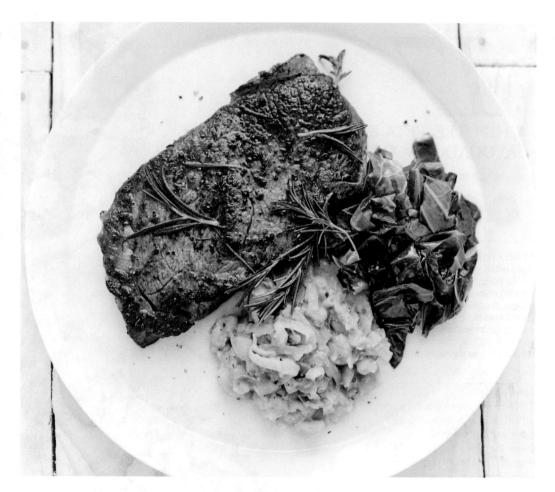

16

ROSEMARY STEAK WITH BEAN MASH

SERVES **4** · CALS **586** · SAT FAT **10.1g** · SUGAR **4g**

INGREDIENTS

2 **rosemary sprigs** · 1 tbsp **balsamic vinegar** · 1 **garlic clove**, crushed · 2 tbsp **olive oil** · 4 **sirloin steaks** (about 120g each), trimmed of fat · 1 **leek**, finely sliced · 2 x 400g cans **cannellini beans**, drained, rinsed · 100ml **chicken stock** · 1 tbsp **wholegrain mustard** · 200g **spring greens**, shredded · 1 tbsp **lemon juice**

METHOD

1 Time to sex up your steak nights. Mix the rosemary, vinegar, garlic and 1 tbsp olive oil. Rub into the steaks and leave to marinate. Heat another ½ tbsp oil in a pan and sauté the leek for 5 mins, add the beans, stock and simmer for 2 mins. Mash with the mustard.

2 Get a frying pan smoking hot. Wipe the marinade from the steaks and cook for 2 mins on each side; set aside to rest.

3 Wipe the pan, add ½ tbsp oil and fry the greens for 3 mins. Season and squeeze over the lemon juice then serve with the steak and mash. Now feel free to feast.

17

CHIPOTLE, FETA & AVOCADO TACOS

SERVES 4 · **CALS** 596 · **SAT FAT** 5.8g · **SUGAR** 5.9g

INGREDIENTS
½ **red onion** · juice and zest of 2 **limes** · ¼ tsp **honey** · 1 tbsp **avocado oil** · 6 **spring onions**, chopped · 1 **green pepper**, deseeded, chopped · 1 tbsp **chipotle paste** · 2 x 400g can **black beans** · 400g can **sweetcorn** · 1 **jalapeño chilli**, sliced · 100g **feta**, crumbled · 1 **avocado**, chopped · 4 **corn tortillas**, toasted

METHOD
1 Slice the red onion and put in a bowl with the lime juice, salt and honey. Leave it to marinate until it's pink.
2 Heat the oil in a frying pan, add the spring onions and pepper and sauté 5 mins until soft. Add the paste and beans and cook another 5 mins, stir in the corn, chilli and half the feta until warm. Season with lime juice and zest, stir in the avocado.
3 Pile onto toasted tortillas, top with the pickled onion and crumble feta over. Eat!

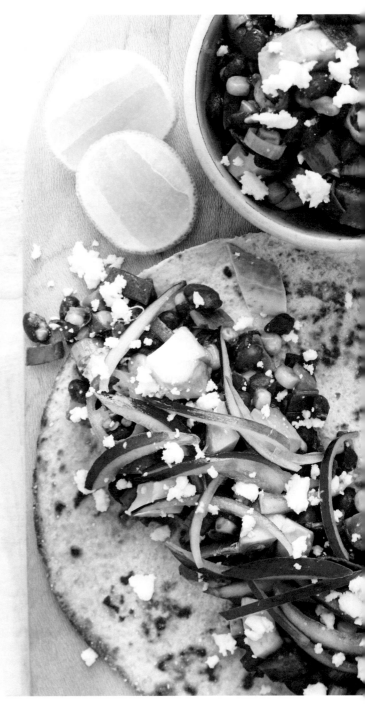

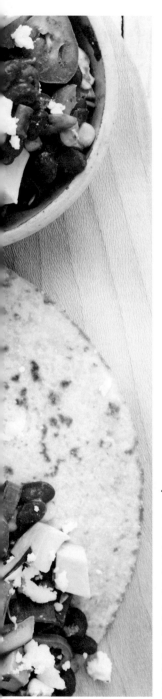

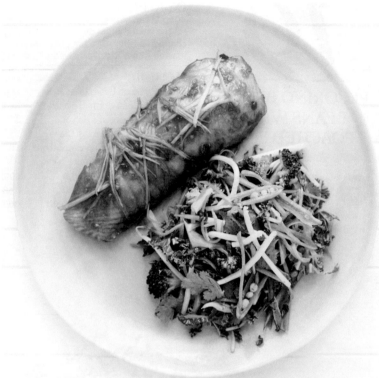

18

SOY SALMON & SLAW

 SERVES **4** CALS **317** SAT FAT **2.7g** SUGAR **9.9g**

INGREDIENTS
4 **salmon fillets** • 2 tbsp **light soy sauce** • 2 tbsp **sweet chilli sauce** • 20g **ginger**, cut into sticks • 100g **kale**, leaves finely shredded • 100g **broccoli florets** • 200g **sugar snap peas**, shredded • 1 **carrot**, shredded • handful **coriander** • handful **bean sprouts** • 2 tbsp **lime juice** • 2 tsp **honey** • 2 tsp **toasted sesame oil**

METHOD
1 Preheat the oven to 200°C. Tear 4 large pieces of foil and place a salmon fillet in each. So far, so good.
2 Now mix the soy sauce, sweet chilli and ginger and spoon over each of the fillets. Wrap the foil loosely around the salmon, sealing the edges tightly. Place on a baking tray and pop in the oven for 12 mins.
3 Now pimp your kale. Cut out the tough stems and finely shred the leaves. Break the broccoli florets into little pieces and toss both with the remaining ingredients. Serve the slaw with the salmon, spooning over any cooking juices. It's all gravy.

19

PECORINO BROAD BEANS WITH POACHED EGG

SERVES	CALS	SAT FAT	SUGAR
4	370	6.2g	3.6g

INGREDIENTS

400g **broad beans** · 50g **grated pecorino** · juice and zest of ½ **lemon** · 3 tbsp **extra-virgin olive oil** · 1 tbsp chopped **flat-leaf parsley** · 1 tbsp chopped **basil** · 1 tbsp chopped **oregano** · 4 slices **rye sourdough**, toasted · 1 **garlic clove**, halved · 4 large **free-range eggs**

METHOD

1 Podding broad beans takes time, but is more than worth it. Blanch the podded beans in a pan of boiling water for 2-3 mins. Drain, cool under cold running water, then slip off and discard the outer skins.
2 Crush the beans in a large pestle and mortar or potato masher. Stir through the grated cheese, lemon juice and zest and 2 tbsp oil, folding in the herbs at the end.
3 Toast the bread, rub with the cut side of the garlic and drizzle with the remaining oil. Pile on the beans. Poach the eggs, and place on top with a splash more oil and a good grind of seasoning. Look at that!

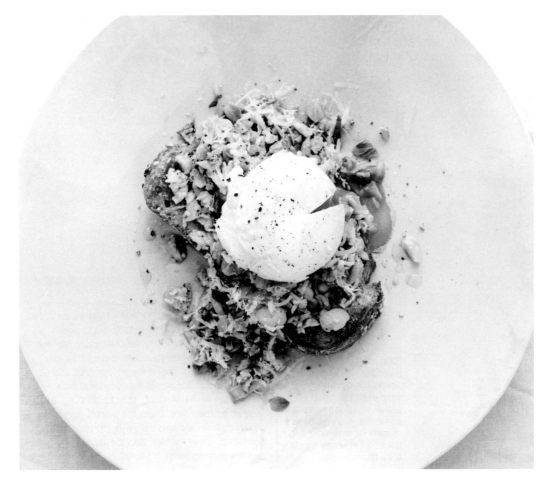

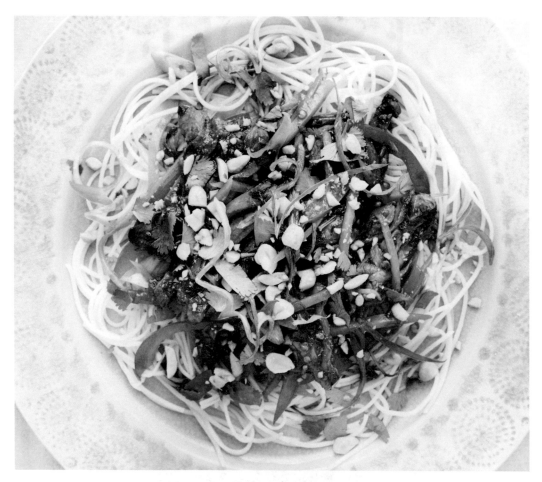

20

KOREAN CHICKEN & GLASS NOODLES

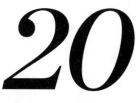

 SERVES **4**   CALS **519**   SAT FAT **3.2g**   SUGAR **12.6g**

INGREDIENTS

4 **skinless and boneless chicken thighs** (500g), cut into strips • 2 tbsp **soya sauce** • 2 tbsp **chilli bean paste** • 2 tbsp **apple cider vinegar** • 2 **garlic cloves**, crushed • 2 tbsp **honey** • 1 tbsp **groundnut oil** • 2 **carrots**, cut into matchsticks • 1 **red pepper**, cut into strips • 6 **spring onions**, sliced • 1 tsp **toasted sesame oil** • 300g **glass noodles**, cooked • handful **peanuts**, toasted, chopped • handful **coriander**

METHOD

1 Put the chicken in a bowl with the soya sauce, chilli bean paste, vinegar, garlic and honey.
2 Heat the groundnut oil in a wok until it's smoking hot. Lift the chicken from the marinade and stir-fry for 4-5 mins until it's golden and charred, then transfer to a plate.

Add a splash more oil to the wok, then throw in the remaining veg. Stir-fry for 2 mins, then tip in any leftover marinade.
3 Toss the chicken and vegetables with the sesame oil, then pile on top of the noodles and scatter with the peanuts and coriander. Now, just add chopsticks.

USE YOUR NOODLE

Vibrant, fresh and bursting with flavours, these one-bowl Vietnamese wonders will leave you satisfied and keep your weightloss on track

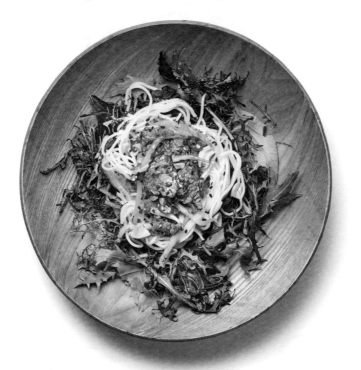

BOUNTIFUL BEEF RICE NOODLES

Serves 2 | 314 cals
0.1g sat fat | 6.9g sugar
20 mins

INGREDIENTS

- 100g **rice noodles** • 200g **mixed salad** • 1 tsp **oil** • 100g **beef fillet**, sliced • 1 tsp chopped **garlic**
- 100ml **stock** • 50g **bean sprouts**
- 2 tbsp **nuoc cham** (mix 1 tsp **rice wine vinegar**, 2 tbsp **fish sauce**, 3 tsp **sugar**, 60ml **water** then boil. Cool, add 1 tsp chopped **garlic** and 1 tsp **lime juice**) • 80g **coriander**
- 2 **chillies** • handful **peanuts**

METHOD

Boil the noodles, then chuck on top of the salad. In a pan, heat the oil then add the beef and garlic, stirring till cooked. Add stock, scraping the pan to make a brown sauce. Stir in bean sprouts, add nuoc cham. Spoon the beef, sprouts and juices into bowls. Garnish with chillies and peanuts. That's it, you're done.

Dish up: Garlic and coriander combine to make a de-bloat dream team. Cheer them on!

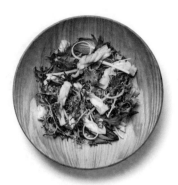

ZESTY CALAMARI CHILLI SALAD

Serves 2 | 80 cals | 0.2g sat fat | 12.7g sugar | 25 mins

• 100g whole **squid**, washed • 5g **ginger**, shredded • 5g **onion**• 5g **celery**, shredded • **chilli marinade** (2 tbsp **lime juice**, 2 tbsp **fish sauce**, ½ tbsp **sugar** and 2 **chillies**,) • 200g **mixed salad** • 1 tbsp **basil leaves**

Cut the squid open lengthways, wash, then score with criss-cross cuts. Next, blanch in boiling water for 30 seconds, then shock it in an ice bath. Drain, pat dry and season. Add ginger, onion, celery and marinade. Let it sit for 15 mins. Arrange the salad in a bowl, top with squid. Garnish with basil. **Dish up:** One squid portion is 90% of your copper RDA, which helps you absorb iron. Legend.

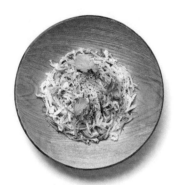

CRUNCHY RADISH SALAD

Serves 2 | 80 cals | 0g sat fat | 8.45g sugar | 10 mins

• 1 **carrot**, sliced into matchsticks • 300g **white radish**, thinly sliced • ½ tsp **salt** • 1 tsp **sugar** • **Chinese cabbage**, thinly sliced • 3 **spring onions** • **chilli powder** • 2 tsp **rice vinegar** • **coriander**, to garnish

Place each of the sliced vegetables in separate bowls. Add salt and sugar to each bowl and let it sit for 5 mins. Press the water out of the carrots and radish, then add the cabbage and spring onion. Add the chilli powder and rice vinegar, and toss. Let it sit for 2 hours. Then garnish... and voilà! **Dish up:** Radish is rich in potassium, for post-workout muscle recovery.

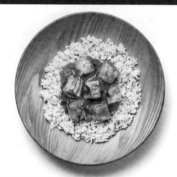

TUCK-IN-QUICK TOMATO TOFU RICE

Serves 2 | 380 cals | 7.8g sat fat' | 6.45g sugar | 35 mins

• 225ml **vegetable oil** • 400g firm **tofu**, cubed • 3 ripe **tomatoes**, chopped • ½ tsp **cane sugar** • ¼ tsp **salt** • 2½ tbsp **fish sauce** • 4 tbsp thinly sliced **spring onions** • 3 tbs shredded **coriander**

Fry the tofu in a frying pan until crisp. Then drain on kitchen paper. Pour out most of the oil from the pan. Return to heat. Add tomatoes, sugar, salt and sauce. Sauté until the tomatoes break down. Pour in 175ml water and simmer. Add tofu and simmer uncovered until liquid has evaporated. Add onions to wilt. Serve with rice and coriander. **Dish up:** Fish sauce is full of the antioxidant glutamic acid, which combats fat storage. Yes!

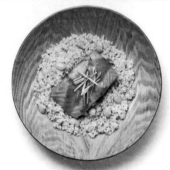

STICKY SALMON BOWL

Serves 2 | 500 cals | 1.5g sat fat| 12g sugar | 25 mins

• 170g **quinoa** • 50g **edamame** • ½ tsp **salt** • 2 tbsp **oil** • tsp **peppercorns** • 2 tbsp **caramel sauce** • knob **ginger**, sliced • 2 x 150g **salmon fillets** • 3 tbsp **fish sauce**

Add quinoa and edamame, salt and 1⅔ cups of water to a saucepan. Bring to the boil then reduce heat to low, cover and cook for 15 mins. Heat oil in a pot, then add peppercorns, caramel and ginger. Lower the heat, place the salmon in the pot, and cover for 8 mins. Plate up with quinoa and pour remaining sauce on top. **Dish up:** A serving of edamame has 37% of your RDA of protein, to stop you snacking.

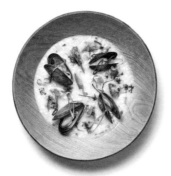

VELVETY SEAFOOD CONGEE

Serves 2 | 304 cals | 1.2g sat fat | 0.5g sugar | 1 hour+

• 3 litres **water** • 200g **broken rice** • 240g **mixed seafood** • 2 tsp **salt** •
2 tbsp **soy sauce** • 2 tsp **shallot oil** • 12g **spring onion** • 12g **shiso**

Put the water in a pot, add rice, bring to boil, then simmer, stirring constantly. Cook for 1 hour until the grains are almost a purée. Add the seafood and mix well. Season with salt, soy sauce and shallot oil. Garnish with spring onion and shiso (an aromatic Japanese herb). **Dish up:** Mussels are rich in DHAs and EPAs – fatty acids that boost brain function.

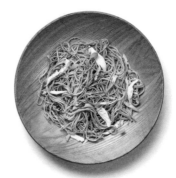

QUICK-SMART CHICKEN NOODLES

Serves 2 | 434 cals | 1.7g sat fat | 2.7g sugar | 15 mins

• 400g **egg noodles** • 3 tbsp **soy sauce** • **vegetable oil** • 3 tbsp
Chinese wine • 2 tbsp **Worcestershire sauce** • 250g **shredded cooked chicken** • 3 **spring onions** • 50g **coriander**

Blanch the noodles in hot water, rinse in cold then drain. Season the noodles with soy sauce and oil then stir in a non-stick pan until they go a little crispy (at around 7 mins). Let the noodles swim in the wine and Worcestershire before adding the chicken and onions. Make it pretty with coriander. **Dish up:** Spring onions contain immune-boosting vitamin A in spades.

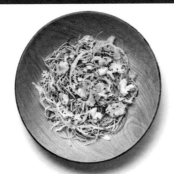

COOL CRAB AND CABBAGE SALAD

Serves 2 | 119 cals | 0g sat fat | 13g sugar | 10 mins

• 50g **white cabbage**, thinly sliced • 50g **carrot**, finely cut • 1 tbsp finely chopped **mint** • 150g cooked **crab meat** • *Dressing:* 50g **caramel** • 10g **lime juice** • 90g water • 5g **red chilli**, minced • 2g **garlic**, minced

As simple as tipping everything into a bowl and mixing, first place the cabbage, carrot and mint in a bowl and mix well. Then place the crab meat in a large mixing bowl with the others. Add the dressing and toss thoroughly. Yep, that's really it. Guaranteed to impress the mother-in-law. **Dish up:** Cabbage is packed full of fibre, which helps keep you slim even when piling on seconds. Oh hello, bikini – long time no see.

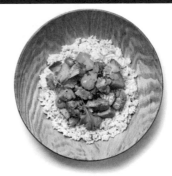

COCO-NUTTY CHICKEN CURRY

Serves 2 | 225 cals | 5.9g sat fat | 6.3g sugar | 35 mins

• 6 **lemongrass stalks** • ½ **onion**, sliced • 1 tbsp **garlic**, chopped • 1 tbsp **ginger** • 5 tbsp **grape seed oil** • 3 tbsp **curry powder** • 1 tsp **chilli powder** • 2 **chicken thighs**, cubed • 2 **carrots**, diced • 125ml **coconut milk**

Start by puréeing lemongrass, onions, garlic and ginger to a paste. Put 3 tbsp oil in a pot on medium heat, stir in paste, curry and chilli. Sauté the chicken until browned, then remove. Add 1 litre water and carrots, cook 20 mins. Add chicken and cook 8 mins. Stir in coconut milk. Serve with rice. **Dish up:** Lemongrass is great for lowering cholesterol, reducing your risk of a stroke or heart disease. Make ours a double.

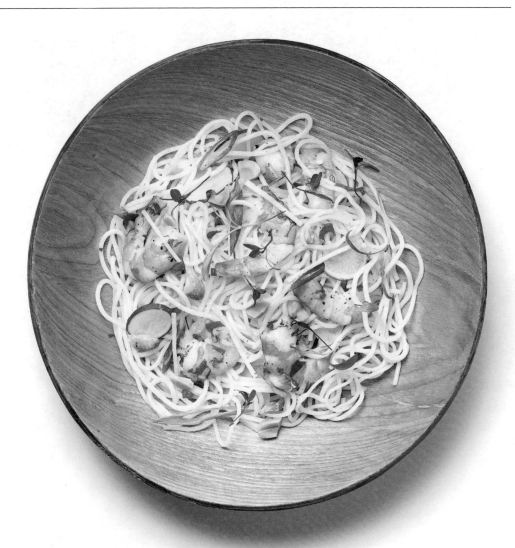

FIERY PRAWN STAR NOODLE BOWL

Serves 2 | 212 cals
0.5g sat fat | 7.7g sugar
20 mins

INGREDIENTS

- 200g **prawns**, peeled • 1 tbsp **ginger**, chopped • 1 tbsp **fish sauce** • 100g **rice noodles** • 50g **radish**, thinly sliced • 50g **spring onions**, sliced • **chilli coconut dressing** (mix 2 tsp chopped **red chillies**, 3 tbsp **coconut sugar**, 1 tbsp **rice vinegar**, 3 tbsp **lime juice**, 1½ tbsp **fish sauce**) • 50g **coriander** • handful **cashews**

METHOD

In a bowl, toss prawns with ginger and fish sauce. Cook noodles, place in a bowl with radish. Cook prawns in a wok with 1 tbsp oil. Add onions for 1 min. Transfer the prawns to the bowl, drizzle over dressing. Garnish with coriander and cashews. **Dish up:** Ginger can help to reduce period pain as much as ibuprofen. It's a monthly godsend.

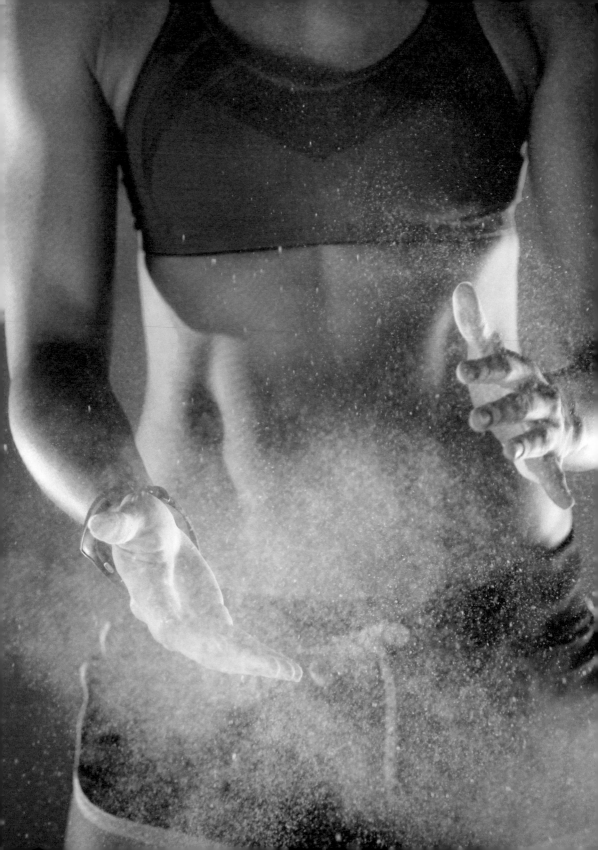

UPGRADE
YOUR
WORKOUT

Spend less time in the gym – and shift fat faster

Here's the good news: the secret to a hotter body is to sweat smarter, not harder, and, in many cases, for shorter durations. In fact, a study from McMaster University in Hamilton, Ontario, found that people who did brief, fast-paced workouts for a total of 90 minutes a week got just as fit as those who did lower-intensity training for four hours and 30 minutes. That gives you an extra three hours a week to play with. But not all short-and-sweet workouts are created equal. This chapter is packed with smarter workout strategies and simple time-saving solutions – to help you unleash your hottest body ever.

START
SMART

S o, first things first. Warm up or not? If you can barely carve out a 30-minute workout window, there's a good chance you'll just skip it. Who wants to waste valuable calorie-torching minutes on tedious knee hugs and neck rolls?

But the reality is that this short-term investment pays off, even if the subsequent sweat-session is only minutes long – as long as you do it right. The best approach involves dynamic stretching, which increases flexibility, improves blood flow, and decreases your risk of injury and recovery time. So, even if your brain is saying 'bring it on!', your muscles aren't ready to work when you first hit the gym. Your central nervous system, which controls movement and activity, is basically in 'power save' mode – and you can blame that on a day at your desk. Before you jump into a workout, your brain needs to signal to your body that it's time for quick, explosive activity.

Warming up can, and usually should, be swift. 'In as few as three minutes, you can increase blood flow and range of motion, improve mental performance, and reduce the risk of injury,' says Andrea Fradkin, PhD, associate professor of exercise science at Bloomsburg University in Pennsylvania. But avoid drawn-out pre-sessions. A study in the US *Journal of Applied Physiology* found that lengthy warm-ups can fatigue you, compromising your actual workout.

There are three crucial steps to an efficient, dynamic warm-up. The warm-up grid (opposite) shows you how to put them to work in a way that best suits the workout that follows. Try to pick movements that mimic what you're about to do – maybe leg swings before a run or walking lunges before strength training.

WARM UP, WARM UP

For a winning warm-up, pick an exercise from each column below and do it for one minute. Choose a different set of three exercises before each workout – you've plenty of choice here. Turn the page for full exercise instructions.

A TURN IT ON	**B UP THE ANTE**	**C PUSH FURTHER**
Kick your nervous system into gear by calling your coordination into action while raising your heart rate and temperature. Now your muscles will respond more effectively during your workout.	This phase turns on underused muscles: glutes, abdominals, hip flexors, and lower- and upper-back muscles. These core muscles maintain stability and control in your joints while you move.	For the finale, you'll increase the range of motion at your joints and improve the flexibility of your large muscle groups. Now you're ready to kick into full-on calorie-burning mode.

A1 CROSS-OVER JUMPING JACKS

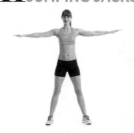

B1 SLOW-MOTION CLIMBER

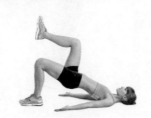

C1 SQUAT TO STAND

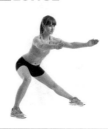

A2 TIGHT CORE ROTATIONS

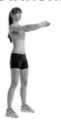

B2 GLUTE BRIDGE MARCH

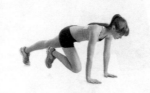

C2 LOW LATERAL LUNGE

A3 HIGH SKIPS

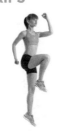

B3 LEG OVERS

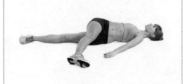

C3 REVERSE LUNGE WITH TWIST

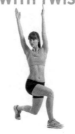

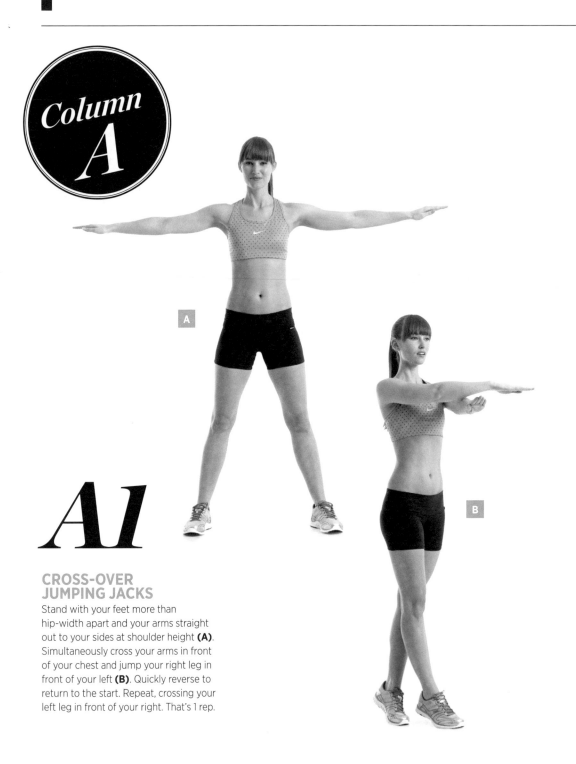

Column
A

A1

CROSS-OVER JUMPING JACKS

Stand with your feet more than hip-width apart and your arms straight out to your sides at shoulder height **(A)**. Simultaneously cross your arms in front of your chest and jump your right leg in front of your left **(B)**. Quickly reverse to return to the start. Repeat, crossing your left leg in front of your right. That's 1 rep.

A2

TIGHT CORE ROTATIONS

Stand with your feet more than hip-width apart and your arms extended in front of you, palms together **(A)**. Keeping your hips and core engaged, rotate your upper body to the right **(B)**. Quickly reverse, twisting all the way to the left. That's 1 rep.

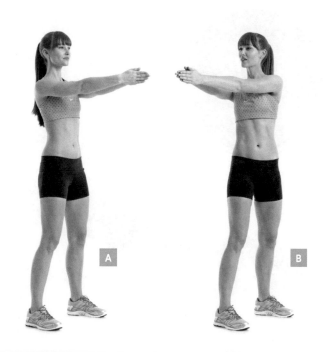

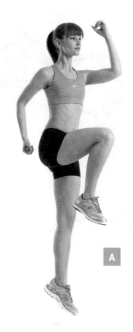

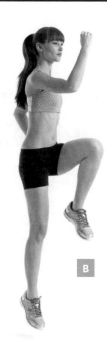

A3

HIGH SKIPS

Skip as high as you can by raising your right knee to hip height and simultaneously raising your left arm **(A)**. Land on the ball of your left foot, then quickly repeat with your opposite arm and leg **(B)**. That's 1 rep.

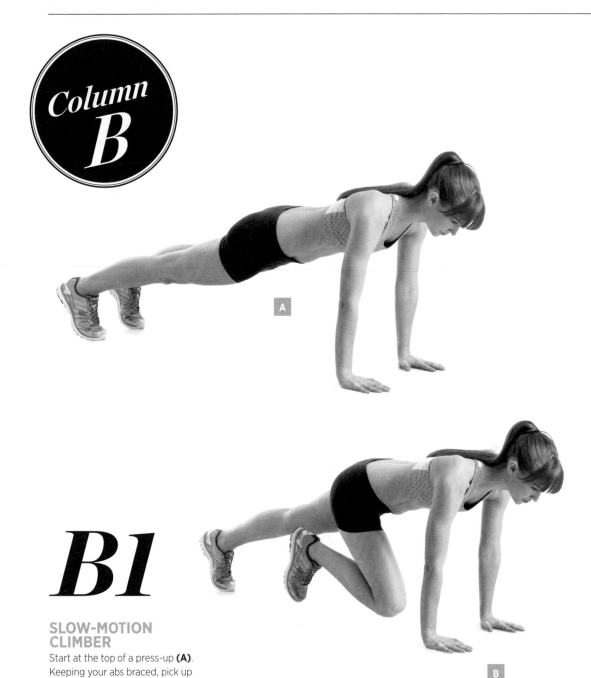

Column B

B1

SLOW-MOTION CLIMBER

Start at the top of a press-up **(A)**. Keeping your abs braced, pick up your right foot and slowly bring your knee toward your right shoulder **(B)**. Hold for 2 seconds, then return to the start. Alternate legs.

B2

GLUTE BRIDGE MARCH

Lie on your back with your knees bent, feet flat on the floor. Raise your hips so your body forms a straight line from shoulders to knees **(A)**. Brace your core and lift your right knee toward your chest **(B)**. Hold for 2 seconds, then lower your right foot. Repeat with the other leg. That's 1 rep.

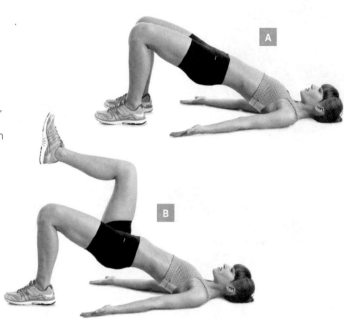

B3

LEG OVERS

Lie face up with your legs straight and arms at your sides **(A)**. Sweep your right leg across your body toward your left hand, keeping your shoulders on the ground **(B)**. Return to the start and switch legs. That's 1 rep.

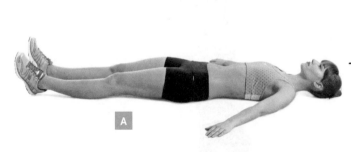

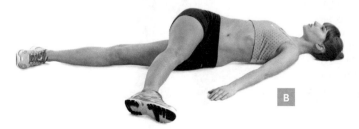

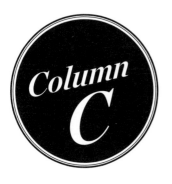

Column **C**

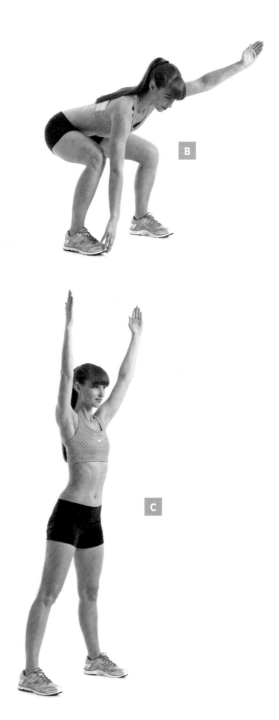

B

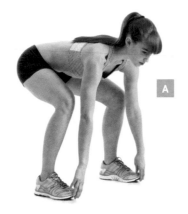

A

C

C1

SQUAT TO STAND

Stand with your feet shoulder-width apart. Keeping your legs straight, bend over and grab your toes. Without letting go of your toes, bend your knees to lower your body into a squat, raising your chest and shoulders **(A)**. Holding that position, raise your left arm directly overhead **(B)**, followed by your right **(C)**. Press through your heels to stand, then lower your arms. That's 1 rep.

C2

LOW LATERAL LUNGE

Step out to the right and bend your knee to lower into a side lunge, keeping your back flat and arms directly out in front of you **(A)**. Without standing, shift to the left, into a lunge on the other side **(B)**. That's 1 rep.

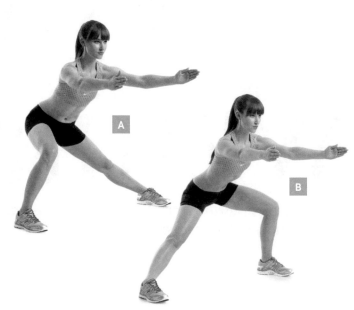

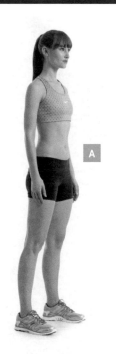
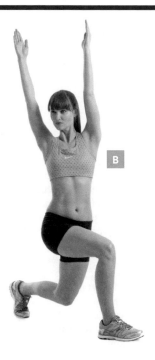

C3

REVERSE LUNGE WITH TWIST

Stand with your feet hip-width apart and your arms at your sides **(A)**. In one motion, step your left foot back and raise your arms overhead, bend both knees to lunge as you twist your shoulders to the right **(B)**. Reverse the movement to return to start. Repeat on the other side.

LOSE YOUR
FEAR OF LIFTING
WEIGHTS

Trade a weekly cardio workout for a strength-training session and you'll see waist-whittling results far quicker

Lifting weights may be the single most efficient way to score a slimmer, sexier body. It also gives you an edge over belly fat, stress, heart disease and cancer. So why aren't more of us doing it?

MYTH *1*
Cardio burns more calories

Experts used to think that aerobic exercise burned more calories than pumping iron. It feels true – not every trip to the weights room leaves you drenched and out of breath like a killer spin class does. But it turns out that strength training has more calorie-torching potential than it was given credit for. Researchers at the University of Southern Maine found that completing a circuit of eight moves (taking about eight minutes) can expend 159 to 231 calories. This is about what you'd burn if you ran at a 10-mile-per-hour pace for the same duration.

In fact, the term 'cardio' shouldn't be limited to just aerobic exercise. A study at the University of Hawaii found that circuit training with weights raises your

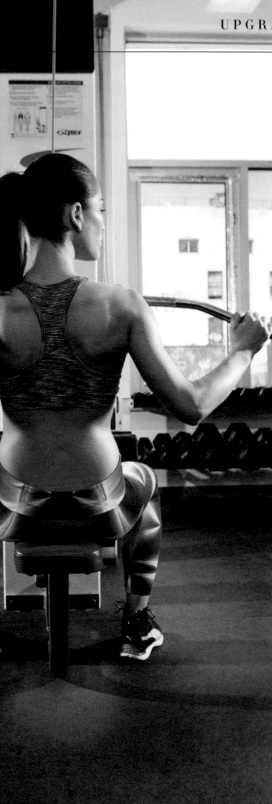

heart rate 15 beats per minute higher than if you ran at 60 to 70% of your max heart rate. The circuit approach provides cardiovascular benefits similar to those of aerobic exercise, while strengthening your muscles – so you save time without sacrificing results.

And if that weren't reason enough, unlike aerobic exercise, the researchers found that a total-body workout with just three big-muscle moves raised participants' metabolisms for 39 hours afterwards. And that means your body will continue to burn calories at a higher rate long after you've kicked off your trainers.

MYTH 2
You can outrun belly fat

Weight training torches body fat better than hours of cardio – plain and simple. In a study at the University of Alabama at Birmingham, one group of dieters lifted three times a week and another did aerobic exercise for the same length of time. Both groups consumed the same number of calories, and both shed the same amount of weight (26lbs). But those who pumped iron dropped 100% fat, whereas the cardio group lost 92% fat and 8% muscle. And this is why that really matters. Muscle loss may drop your scale weight, but it doesn't improve your reflection in the mirror, and it makes you more likely to gain back the flab you lost. But if you strength-train while you diet, you'll build lean muscle mass and burn more fat. Experts estimate that for every three pounds of muscle you build, you can burn an extra 120 calories a day, because muscle takes more energy to sustain. Over the course of a year, that's about 10lbs of fat – without spending more time in the gym or changing your diet.

MYTH 3
Aerobic exercise keeps your heart healthy

Okay, yes, that's true, but cardio isn't the only way to get your blood pumping. Researchers at the University of Michigan found that people who did three total-body weight workouts a week for two months reduced their diastolic blood pressure (the bottom number) by an average of eight points. That's enough to reduce the risk of a stroke by 40% and the chance of a heart attack by 15%.

University of South Carolina researchers found that total-body strength is linked to a reduced risk of death from cardiovascular disease and cancer. Other scientists found that being strong during middle age is associated with "exceptional survival," which is defined as living to 85 without developing a major disease.

MYTH *4*
Lifting makes you bulky

Women often think they shouldn't lift because they want to be toned, long and lean, not bulky. But the fact is that muscles are, by definition, lean and their length is set once our body is mature. No workout can make them leaner in themselves and, outside of surgery, there isn't much you can do to alter their length. In fact, there are only two ways that muscle can go: it can either get bigger or smaller.

Exercisers hoping for 'toned' need to aim for a body fat percentage that's low enough to reveal muscle definition. When you build muscle, but don't attack the body fat that lies on top of it, you may feel bigger and heavier. Conversely, methods like Pilates and yoga typically don't use the same level of resistance, which may mean you won't build as much muscle, so even if your body fat percentage remains the same, you at least don't feel as if you're getting denser. Many of these routines help improve posture, which can give you the appearance of being longer and leaner.

WEIGH YOUR OPTIONS

Lifting too much too soon can affect your form and put you at risk of injury, but using lighter weights won't test your muscles enough. Use this cheat-sheet to gauge starting weights for beginners.

If you're doing...	Start with...
Lateral raises	2½ to 5lbs in each hand
Biceps curls	5 to 8lbs in each hand
Flat-bench dumbbell rows	12 to 20lbs
Chest presses	12lbs (body bar) to 45lbs
Squats	zero (body weight) to 45lbs

These light-resistance methods can actually sabotage your goals in the long run. Research shows that between the ages of 30 and 50, you'll probably lose 10% of your body's total muscle. And it's likely to be replaced by fat. Even participants who maintained their body weight for up to 38 years lost three pounds of muscle and added three pounds of fat each decade.

Why does that matter? Because even if their body weight remained the same, their dress size didn't. Lean muscle mass actually has 18% less volume than a similar amount of body fat. So, building lean muscle mass through strength training is the real secret to revealing a leaner, more toned body.

MYTH *5*
To run better, you must run more

It turns out that extra pavement-pounding isn't the only, or necessarily the most effective, way to become a better runner. The US *Journal of Strength and Conditioning Research* found that runners who did resistance-training exercises two or three days a week, in addition to their weekly cardio, increased their leg strength and enhanced their endurance – two things that improve performance and contribute to weight loss.

Lifting can also keep you injury free. A study in the US journal *Clinical Biomechanics* found that female runners who did six weeks of lower-body exercises improved their leg strength, particularly in the hips – a common source of pain and injury for runners.

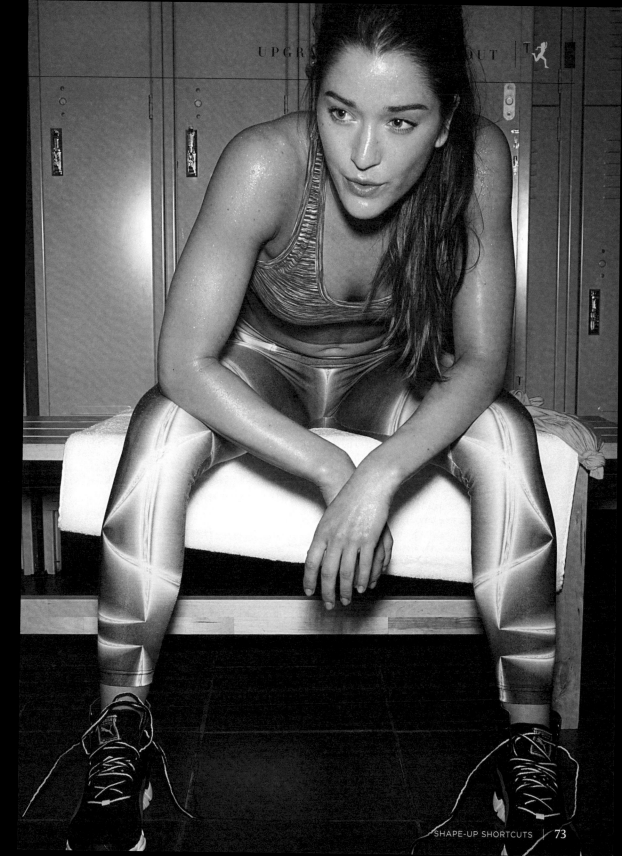

HOW TO
BURN FAT
FASTER
WITH
EIGHTS

It's relatively easy to translate higher intensity into spin class (pedal faster) or on the treadmill (increase the pace), but how do we best increase our efforts during strength-training workouts? Fast-track your results by incorporating these training strategies. Because, what's more impressive than spending an hour in the weights room? Spending just 30 minutes – and getting an even better workout

Watch your speed

In the weights room, tempo training refers to the speed you lift and lower resistance during an exercise, and adjusting it is a great way to get more out of every rep. Sometimes this means moving through exercises more quickly. Researchers have found that exercisers who performed a weight-lifting workout at a quick, explosive pace expended 70 more calories, on average, than those who did the workout at a normal pace.

But you can also score benefits from slowing down your workouts. Your muscle has three main types of contractions: eccentric (lengthening of muscle fibres during the lowering portion of an exercise, like lowering into a squat); isometric (muscle length staying the same while under tension, like the bottom position of a squat) and concentric (the shortening of muscle fibres during the lifting portion of the exercise, like standing up from a squat). Slowing down during the eccentric portion of an exercise can help improve body awareness and stability, as well as stimulate the muscle fibres differently by placing them under more stress. *The Journal of Strength and Conditioning Research* found that an eccentric tempo (taking three seconds) significantly increased the amount of calories that both trained and untrained individuals burned for up to 72 hours post-workout. The slow eccentric phase increases the tension on the muscle, which creates a higher calorie burn during and after exercise in order to repair the muscles.

And, yes, you can even burn calories without moving a muscle. It's called isometric training, after

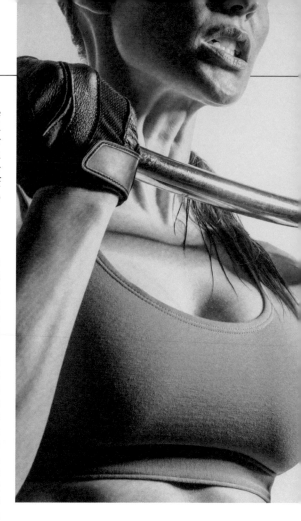

that second muscle contraction where the muscle length stays the same while under tension. Take a wall squat, for example. Your quads are constantly under stress, even though they don't move. This can be an especially useful strategy for people who lack stability or are dealing with injuries. As with other aspects of your workout regime, you should mix up tempos so your body doesn't adapt to the pace.

Lift heavy

Dumbbells, resistance bands, even water – they're all ways to apply external force to your workout to make any routine more challenging. The added stress encourages muscle growth, which helps increase your metabolism and blast fat. But in order to get a tighter, leaner body, the chosen resistance has to actually tax your muscles.

This means saying goodbye to feather-light dumbbells. We're not saying that lifting lighter weights is completely ineffective. Researchers found that lifting 30% of your all-out max can be as effective as 80% of your max – but, here's the important part – as long as you do enough reps to tire out your muscles. It's going to take considerably more reps at a lighter weight to match the effectiveness. But, again, it comes back to your goal. If it is faster fat loss, supersizing your dumbbells is a better use of your gym time. Hoisting heavier weights builds lean muscle in less time, plus research shows you can burn nearly twice as many calories in the two hours after lifting heavier weights.

Use more muscle

Many women, especially if they're new to strength training, stick to a handful of the same exercises – usually biceps curls, calf raises, and crunches. They eventually work a good amount of muscles, head to toe, but it takes a while, since they're only focusing on one muscle group at a time with isolation exercises.

But even if the end goal is simply to look great in a bikini, most of us would benefit from a more athletic training approach. The strength work of athletes places a significant emphasis on movements that we replicate in real life – like squatting, pushing, stepping, jumping, and pulling – rather than just body parts or single muscle groups. Also referred to as 'functional training', these big-body exercises help you move bigger weights and build more muscle. At the same time, this movement-centered approach improves mobility, meaning your muscles and joints are able to withstand the stress placed on them during workouts and throughout each day without getting injured.

But you won't just move better and feel stronger. Targeting multiple muscle groups together (called compound exercises) recruits more muscle fibres,

PHOTOGRAPHY: GETTY IMAGES

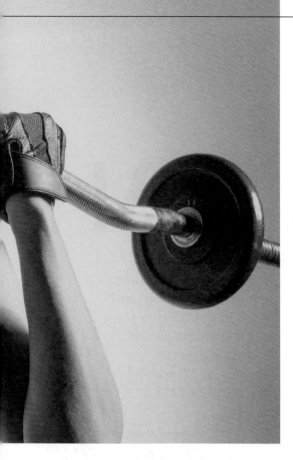

which translates to a higher calorie burn in less time. This functional approach also makes your body a stronger, more efficient unit, so you can challenge it more, which means you'll work it harder and see results faster. Take a look at your workout; no less than 50% of the exercises should be big-body moves, as opposed to isolated (or single-joint) exercises.

Rest less

Walk into any weights room and you'll find a handful of people standing around not doing much that resembles working out. But just because your legs need a break after squats doesn't mean your whole body does. With the right programme, you can take advantage of that downtime by training another muscle group. Take supersets: two exercises that work opposing muscle groups, performed back-to-back without rest – for example, a chest-press combined with a bent-over row. Supersets accomplish more work in a shorter

period of time without compromising the effort of each set. A study in the US *Journal of Strength and Conditioning Research* found that participants burned 33% more calories after doing supersets, compared with sets that let you rest between moves.

Another method that works is circuit training. Moving through a series of strength exercises, going from one to the next with little to no rest, is a simple short cut that cuts your gym time in half, without cutting corners on your results. What's more, minimising your downtime between moves also keeps your heart rate elevated and helps maximise the fat-burning impact of your workout.

Power up

Muscle strength isn't the only thing that can jump-start a sluggish metabolism. Muscle power (sometimes referred to as speed-strength by trainers) is about generating as much force as fast as possible, and it can be a useful weight-loss tool.

Workouts that incorporate explosive movements, commonly called plyometrics, are one of the most effective ways to torch calories and burn serious fat. They also fire up your fitness level by improving your coordination and agility. They can even boost your speed. Researchers at the University of Nebraska found that participants who improved their vertical jump also logged significantly faster 10K running times.

Whether they're jumps or quick upper-body movements, plyometric exercises increase the elastic properties of your muscles, which, over time, allows them to handle intense workloads more efficiently. The result? Your muscles adapt to more challenging workouts faster, so you see body-shaping results sooner.

Because these types of exercises can be higher impact and harder on your joints, ease into them slowly. When starting a new plyo routine, only do it once a week for the first two weeks.

FIX YOUR FORM

If you've been going to the gym regularly but not seeing great results, it may be because you're mangling your moves. Experts agree that proper form is the single most important factor in injury prevention, yet many women don't give it a lot of thought – especially when we're in a rush

Most of us make tiny but key errors in our techniques, and these mistakes will prevent us from building muscle and burning more calories. Regardless of what pace you're moving at, you never want to train at a speed that compromises control. When any workout cranks up the intensity or speed, quality can take a back seat to quantity. People sometimes get so focused on banging out as many reps as they can, however they can – even if it means sacrificing form. While the occasional slam of a weight stack is par for the course when using resistance equipment like the cable machine, lowering the weight without control can result in injury. It can also prevent you from getting the results you're after, because you don't work through the full range of motion. With every exercise, make sure your primary objective is proper form – you can worry about picking up speed later.

The four basic moves on the next two pages can trip women up. Apply these form fixes to upgrade your routine – and your body.

QUICK TIP

A good strategy for first-timers is to do all the exercises without any resistance first. Going through the movement pattern with proper form – but no heavy weights – helps teach your body and brain how to move correctly.

1

LUNGES

Main mistake: You lean forward, causing your front heel to rise.

Narrow your starting stance. The closer your feet are, the harder your core has to work to stabilise your body **(A)**.

As you do the lunge, focus on moving your torso only up and down, not pushing it forward. This keeps your weight balanced evenly through your front foot, allowing you to press into the floor with your heel, which tones more lower-body muscles **(B)**.

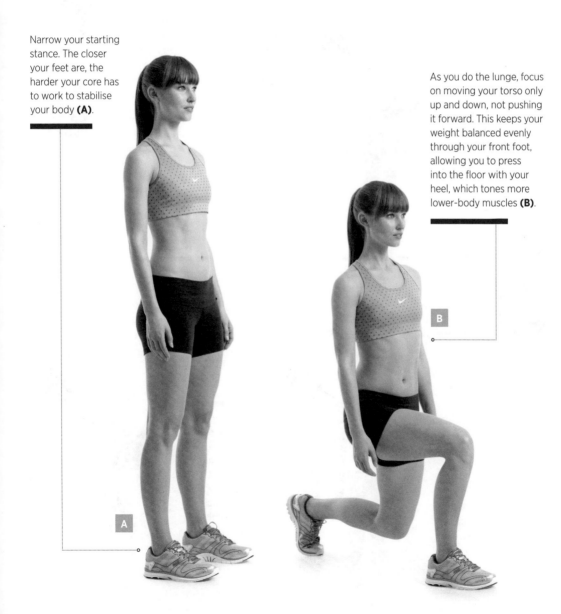

2

STRAIGHT-LEG DEADLIFTS
Main mistake: You round your lower back as you bend over.

It's easy to put too much space between the weight and your body as you move up and down. Pretend you're shaving your legs with the bar or dumbbells. The further the weights are from your body, the more strain on your back, which limits the work of your hamstrings and glutes.

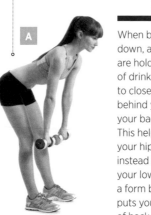

When bending down, act as if you are holding a tray of drinks and need to close the door behind you with your backside **(A)**. This helps you push your hips back instead of rounding your lower back – a form blunder that puts you at risk of back problems.

As you return to standing, squeeze your glutes. You'll engage your bum rather than strain your lower back **(B)**.

3

ROWS AND PULL-UPS
Main mistake: You ignore the muscles that draw back your shoulder blades.

Before you start the exercise, create as much space as you can between your ears and shoulders. Pull your shoulder blades down and back, which will ensure you work the intended middle- and upper-back muscles **(A)**.

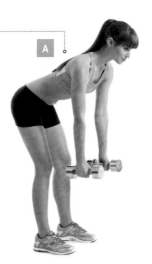

Imagine there is an orange between your shoulder blades. As you pull the weights or your body up, "squeeze the juice out of it" by bringing your shoulder blades together **(B)**.

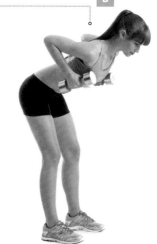

4

SQUATS

Main mistake: You start the movement by bending your knees.

Women tend to lean forward on their toes, but they should sit back into their heels. Try this fix: pretend that you're standing on a paper towel and imagine trying to rip the towel apart by pressing your feet onto the floor and outward **(A)**. This activates your glutes, which helps you break through plateaus.

As you squat, imagine you're sitting down into a chair, rather than forward on top of your knees. Push your hips back first instead of beginning by bending your knees, which puts more stress on your joints **(B)**.

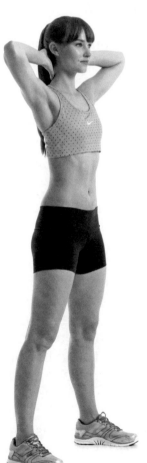

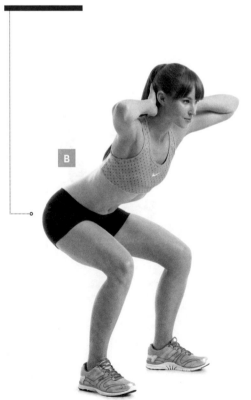

DITCH *THE* MACHINES

Full-body, multi-muscle moves are best achieved using free weights – you'll burn far more calories

Free weights, such as barbells and dumbbells, challenge your body more than machines do. They engage more muscles, increase the range of motion, and are less likely to cause injury. Still, many women spend most of their time at the gym hopping from one exercise machine to the next. The problem is that many machines isolate one muscle, which means you burn fewer calories and work fewer muscles. Try these replacement exercises instead.

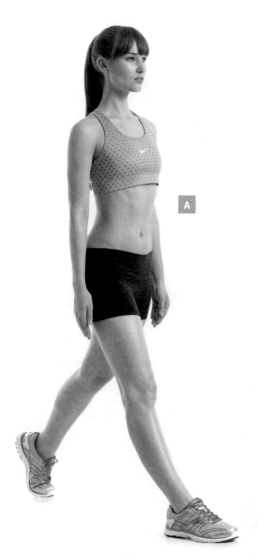

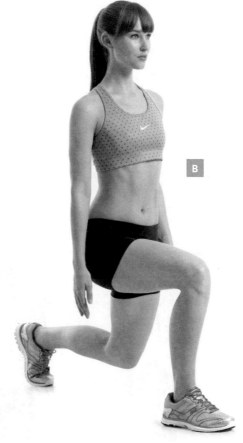

THE MACHINE
SEATED LEG EXTENSION

Sure, you'll strengthen your quads – but at a cost. The resistance is close to your ankle, which puts a high amount of torque on your knee when you raise and lower the weight. The result? Kneecap pain.

THE REPLACEMENT
SPLIT SQUAT

This move puts less stress on your knees, plus it works your hamstrings and glutes. Step one foot 3 to 4 feet in front of the other **(A)**, then bend your knees and lower your back knee toward the floor **(B)**. Press through the heel of the front foot to stand. Do 10 reps, then switch legs.

THE MACHINE
SEATED ABS CRUNCH

Spinal flexion – bending forward as you do during a crunch – is the cause of most back pain. Think of it like a credit card: bend it once and it won't break but bend it 100 times and see what happens. By adding weight, this machine places even more pressure on your spinal discs, increasing the risk of pain and injury.

THE REPLACEMENT
STABILITY-BALL ROLLOUT

Your core is meant to stabilise your spine, not move it, and this exercise engages your entire core to keep your spine neutral. Kneel on the ground and place your forearms on a stability ball, palms together **(A)**. Brace your core and slowly roll the ball away from you, keeping your back flat **(B)**. Slowly pull the ball back to the starting position. That's 1 rep. Work up to 20.

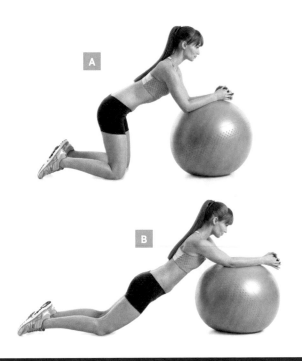

THE MACHINE
BICEPS CURL

The biggest problem here is that it's so easy to cheat! People often rely on gravity to lower (read: drop) the bar, and cutting your range of motion short not only makes the exercise less effective, but also causes muscle tightness and strains your elbows and wrists.

THE REPLACEMENT
BAND-ASSISTED CHIN-UP

This move hits your biceps, back, shoulders, and core, and strengthens the muscles that help you stand tall, so you look longer and leaner. Loop a resistance band around a chinup bar, threading one end through the other and pulling it tightly. Grab the bar with a shoulder-width, underhand grip, place your knee in the loop of the band, and hang at arm's length **(A)**. Pull yourself up to the bar **(B)**. Work up to 10 reps.

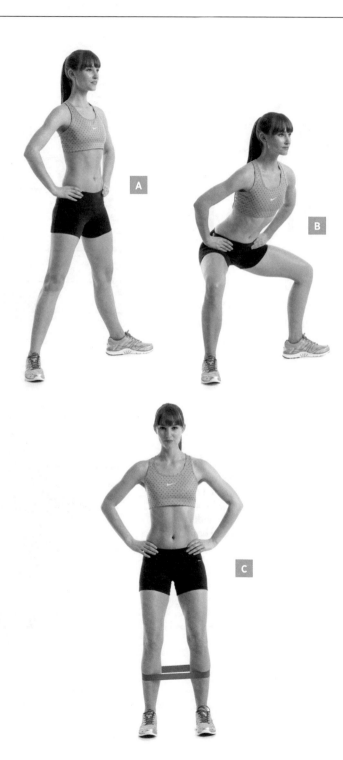

THE MACHINE
HIP ADDUCTOR/ABDUCTOR

Sitting down and squeezing your legs together or pushing them apart won't shrink your thighs, no matter how many reps you bang out. These are nonfunctional, unnatural movement patterns that offer zero payoff. And the abductor move could irritate your iliotibial band, the connective tissue that runs from the outside of your hip to the outside of your knee.

THE REPLACEMENT
PLIÉ SQUAT

Pliés are a far better leg toner because they hit your inner thighs and your quads, hamstrings, and glutes. Stand with your feet wide and turned out 45 degrees **(A)**. Sit your hips back and bend your knees to lower your body until your thighs are nearly parallel to the floor **(B)**. Return to the start. That's 1 rep. Do 3 sets of 10.

LATERAL BAND WALK

Lateral band walks tone the outer thighs, glutes, and hips. Place a small resistance loop around your calves **(C)** and sidestep to the right for 15 feet. Step to the left to return to the starting position. That's 1 set. Repeat twice more.

WORKOUT AT HOME

You can avoid the gym completely if you like. And nor do you need a room full of expensive kit to get into shape. Here are a few of the best pieces to bring home

DUMBBELLS

These are the single most essential workout tool. There are literally hundreds of exercises you can do with dumbbells. If you can, get at least two pairs (one light, one heavy) so that you can mix and match depending on the exercise. Check out One Dumbbell, One Hot Body on page 148.

STABILITY BALL

It's a great tool for core exercises and can also substitute for a bench in some exercises to increase the difficulty and up the core activation.

RESISTANCE BANDS

Big ones can make bodyweight squats extra challenging, or help with assisted chin-ups, while smaller bands are great for waking up the underworked muscles in your hips and bum.

KETTLEBELL

It can be used in the same way as a dumbbell, but because of its unique shape, it's even more versatile. Check out the Ultimate Kettlebell Workout on page 152.

CHIN-UP BAR

Bodyweight exercises cover every basic movement – except pulling. And nothing trains you better than chin-ups.

PHOTOGRAPHY: MANUETAKA TOKUYAMA

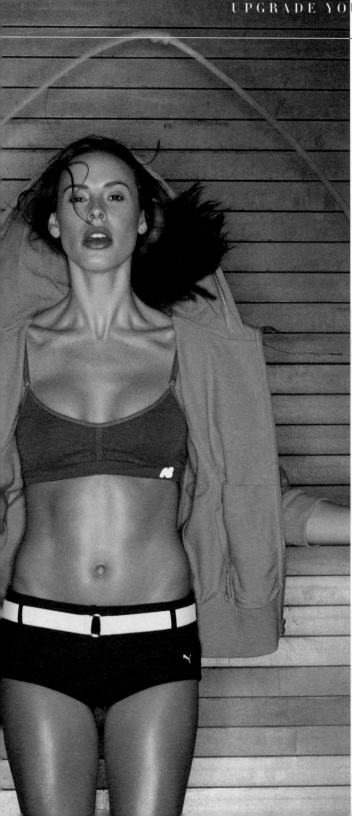

SKIPPING ROPE

A cost-effective, portable, calorie-incinerating tool that's perfect for picking up your heart rate during a warm-up, or spiking your calorie-burn during your workout.

FOAM ROLLER

Soothe sore muscles and loosen tight fascia (the connective tissue that surrounds muscles) for improved recovery, better performance, and a more lithe look. Check out Work Out The Kinks on page 180.

TRX

This suspension trainer leverages your own weight to adjust the resistance of any total-body move. Setup is simple – just flip over a door or around a (sturdy) stair banister – and it packs into a small bag, so you can stash it when you're not using it. Check out Tone Every Inch on page 142.

BENCH, STEP, OR BOX

Adjustable benches add variety to free-weight training. A basic cardio step or box can be a great starting point for beginners wanting to target, triceps, abs, and thighs. Check out Step Up Your Results on page 158.

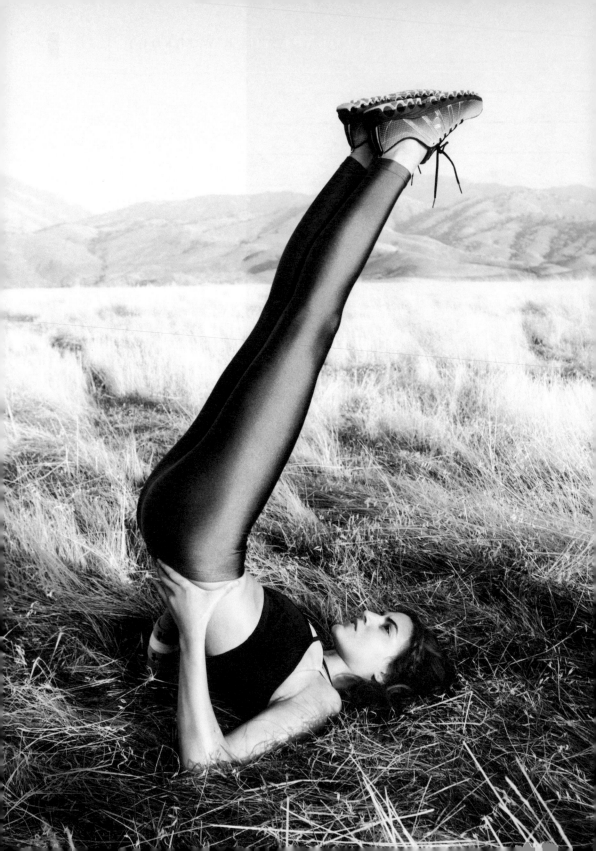

RESHAPE YOUR BODY

The quickest fat-loss plan ever!

A flexible fitness mentality can be an effective way to drop pounds. But while improvising your way through workouts may offer variety, it can also make it harder to develop consistency. The key to creating a sustainable training plan is to address both your strength and cardio needs in short, simple and effective workouts. These two plans blend functional, balanced strength training in a circuit with short rest breaks, to boost the cardiovascular benefits without compromising lean muscle mass – which helps you burn even more calories after your workout. And you'll be done and on your way in 24 minutes.

GET FIT, FAST

Complete three routines each week on non-consecutive days, alternating between Workout A and Workout B (so A-B-A during the first week, B-A-B during the second week, etc). For each workout, start with the first exercise and complete as many reps as you can in 30 seconds, then rest 30 seconds; repeat this pattern until you've completed each move. That's one set. Repeat three more times for a total of four sets – it should take you about 20 minutes. If you're a beginner, or it's been longer than two months since you've last exercised, repeat just one more time for a total of two sets.

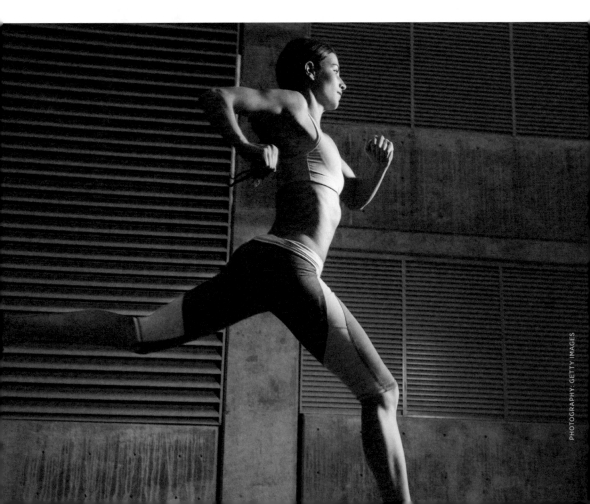

Workout A

1

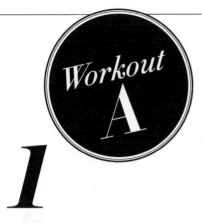
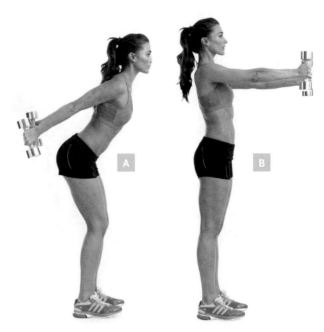

DUMBBELL SKIER SWING

Hold a pair of dumbbells and stand with your feet hip-width apart. Push your hips back and bring the weights behind you **(A)**, then quickly thrust your hips forward and swing the dumbbells to shoulder height **(B)**. That's 1 rep; continue in a fluid, consistent motion.

2

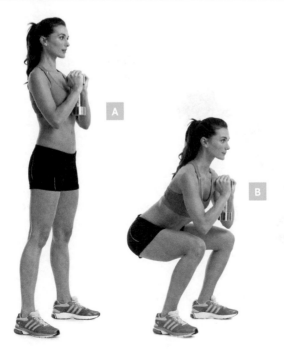

DUMBBELL GOBLET SQUAT

Stand with your feet hip-width apart and hold a dumbbell vertically in front of your chest, with both hands cupping the dumbbell head **(A)**. Push your hips back and bend your knees to lower into a squat **(B)**. Push yourself back to start. That's 1 rep.

3

SUSPENDED PRESS-UP

Secure a TRX, or other suspension system, face away from the anchor point, with your feet shoulder-width apart, and hold both handles in front of your chest, arms extended **(A)**. Bend your elbows to lower your chest toward the handles (doing a press-up), keeping a straight line from head to heels **(B)**. Pause, then press back to the start. That's 1 rep.

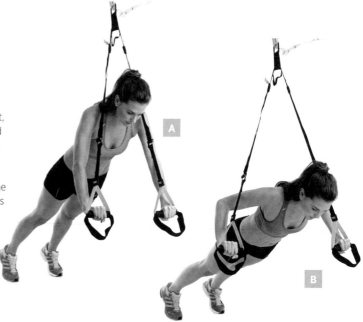

4

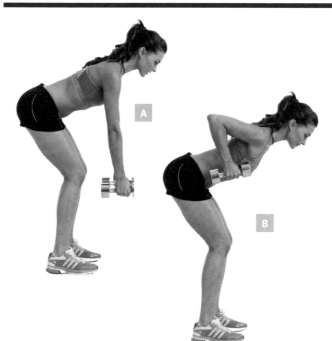

DUMBBELL ROW

Holding a pair of dumbbells, stand with your feet hip-width apart, knees bent, arms hanging straight, palms facing each other; bend forward to lower your torso toward the floor **(A)**. Pull your shoulder blades together and row the weights toward your chest **(B)**. Return to the start. That's 1 rep.

5

BODY SAW

Place your feet on sliding exercise discs (or use paper plates or towels) and get into a press-up position, hands under your shoulders **(A)**. Keeping your body in a straight line from head to heels, push your feet away from you as far as you can **(B)**. Pull back to start. That's 1 rep.

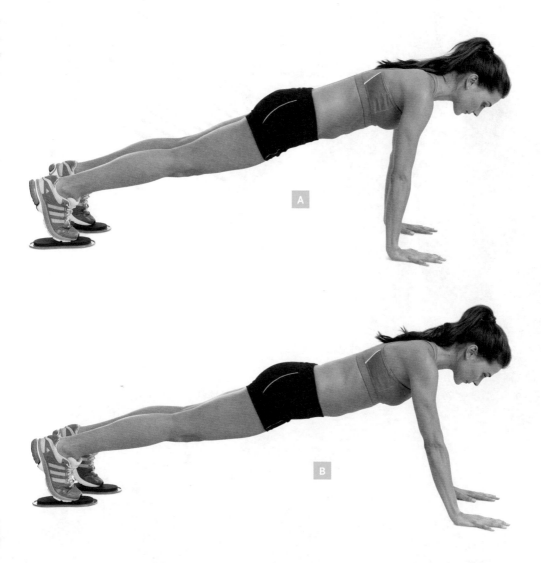

A

B

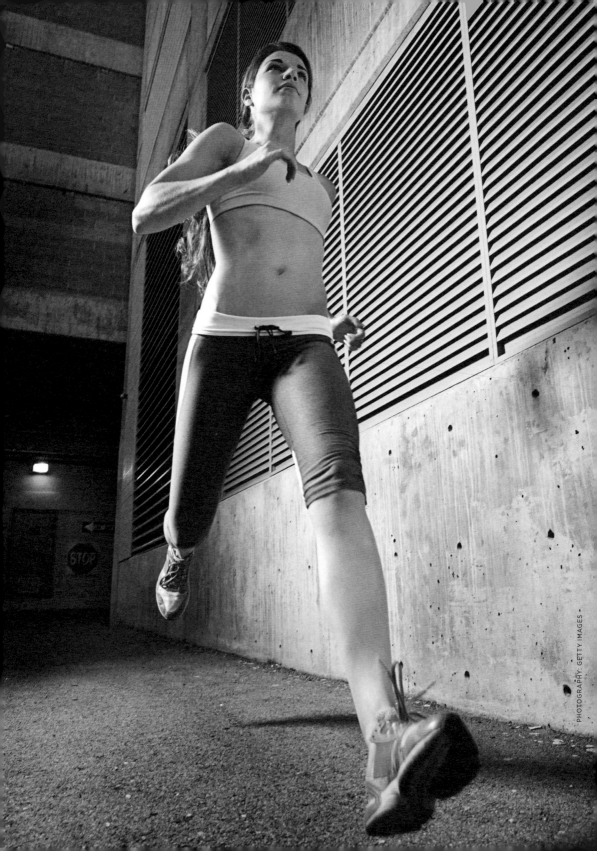

Workout **B**

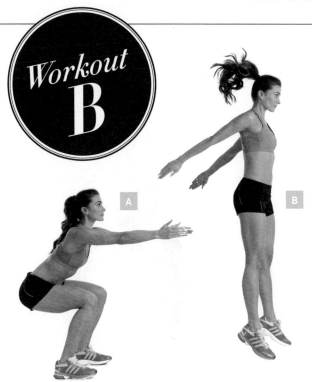

1

JUMP SQUAT

Standing with your feet hip-width apart, sit your hips back to lower into a squat, raising your arms in front of you at shoulder height **(A)**. Press through your heels to jump as high as you can off the ground, swinging your arms behind you **(B)**. That's 1 rep. Land softly and immediately lower into your next squat.

2

WALKING LUNGE

Stand with your feet hip-width apart, hands on your hips **(A)**. Step forward with your left leg and lower your body until both knees are bent 90 degrees **(B)**. Press through your left heel and bring your right foot forward as you return to standing. That's 1 rep. Repeat on the other side and continue alternating.

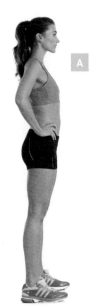

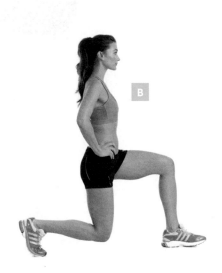

3

DUMBBELL PUSH PRESS

Hold a pair of dumbbells at shoulder height, palms facing each other, feet hip-width apart. Bend your knees slightly **(A)**, then stand and press the dumbbells overhead, straightening your arms completely **(B)**. That's 1 rep.

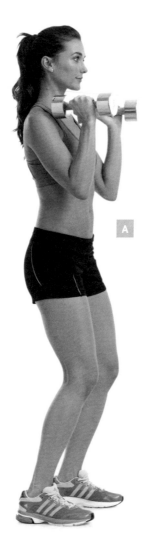

A

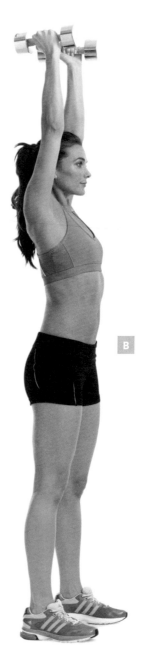

B

SUSPENDED ROW

Secure a TRX or other suspension system and face the anchor point, holding both handles in front of your chest, arms straight, feet shoulder-width apart **(A)**. Keep your shoulders back; bend your elbows to pull your body toward the anchor point **(B)**. Pause, then slowly return to start. That's 1 rep.

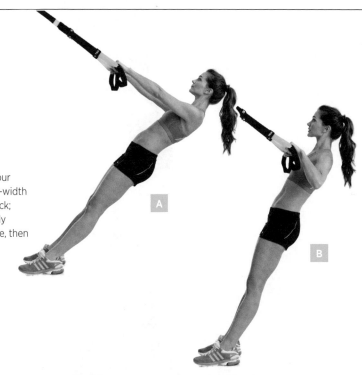

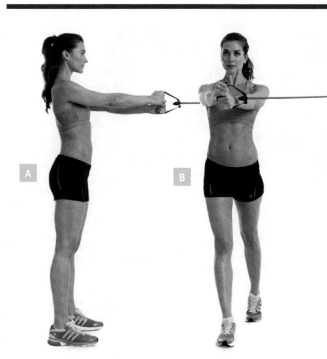

ALTERNATING BAND ROTATIONS

Stand facing a resistance band (secured a few feet away from you at chest height) and grab the handle with both hands, then step away until you feel tension **(A)**. Brace your core and pull the handle to the right while rotating your hips and shoulders **(B)**. Pause, then return to start. That's 1 rep. Repeat on the left side.

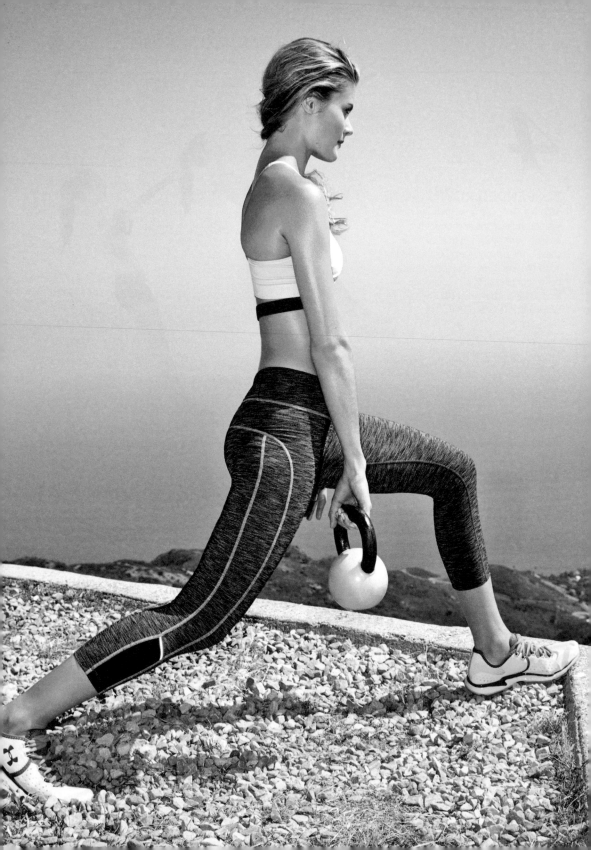

5-MINUTE
FAT
FIXES

Turbocharge your metabolism and get fit fast

Even if we could all find five free minutes each day (and actually, who can't?), most of us wouldn't use the time to work out. We assume that's not long enough to achieve anything significant. Then there's the simple truth that not many workouts are created for super-short time-frames. So, the virtuous few with an anything-is-better-than-nothing attitude do a few minutes of crunches, press-ups and lunges while they watch TV. Better than nothing? Sure. But there's so much more you can achieve. These workouts deliver maximum results in minimum time – no matter how busy you are.

MAXIMISE
EVERY MINUTE

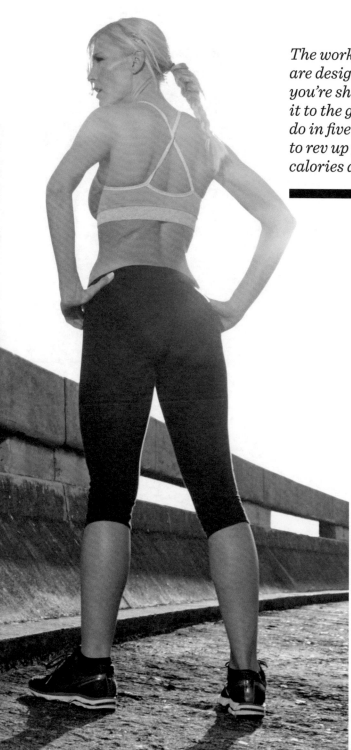

The workouts in this chapter are designed for those days when you're short on time or can't make it to the gym. Five exercise you can do in five minutes: that's all it takes to rev up your metabolism, torch calories and sculpt muscle

These workouts are intentionally minimal. They're perfect for the days when you're tired or demotivated. You won't need anything more than dumbbells (two pairs, one heavy and one light) and a box, bench, or step and you can adapt them to your needs. They can be used as a workout in between sessions of your regular strength regime – when your schedule is just too hectic, committing to five minutes is an efficient and effective way to maintain consistency. And when you're not pressed for time, you can repeat the same workout three to five times for a full-length circuit workout. They make great back-pocket plans, for when you get to the gym with no fixed idea and need something effective and easy to remember. Or mix and match a few of the workouts for a longer session that has a wider variety of moves.

Just like sprints on a treadmill or in spin class, you have to push hard and fast the entire time. That's what helps dial up the calorie burn and leaves a lingering impression on your metabolism. But while plenty of exercises can leave your lungs burning and muscles aching in the same amount of time, these moves are designed so that, when paired

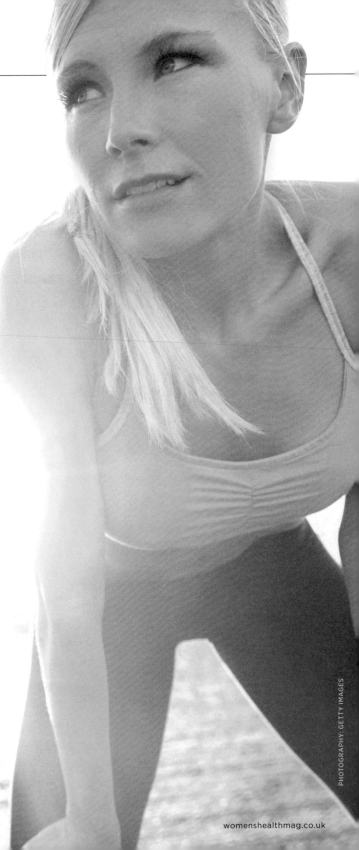

together, they'll give you an effective and balanced total-body workout. Not only will they build strength and work your major muscle groups, they will also help develop rotational strength, core stability, hip mobility, and overall flexibility. And that means that, in as little as five minutes, these workouts will help you build functional, balanced strength – and, of course, kick-start your fat burners.

Interval exchange

Pick one of these two intervals to complete any of the following workouts. Both burn calories and blast fat, but each generates a slightly different metabolic response. Switching between them not only helps speed up results, it also offers enough variety to fight mental fatigue.

30:30 Complete as many reps as you can in 30 seconds, then rest for 30 seconds before moving on to the next exercise. (Rest 60 seconds at the end if you're doing more than one round.) Choose the heaviest weights, that will allow you to work for the entire time and maintain proper form, but challenge you to complete the set.

50:10 Complete as many reps as you can in 50 seconds, then rest for 10 seconds before moving on to the next exercise. (Rest 60 seconds at the end if you're doing more than one round.) You'll need to use lighter weights, but because you'll be able to perform more reps, it should still feel as tough to finish a set.

Workout *1*

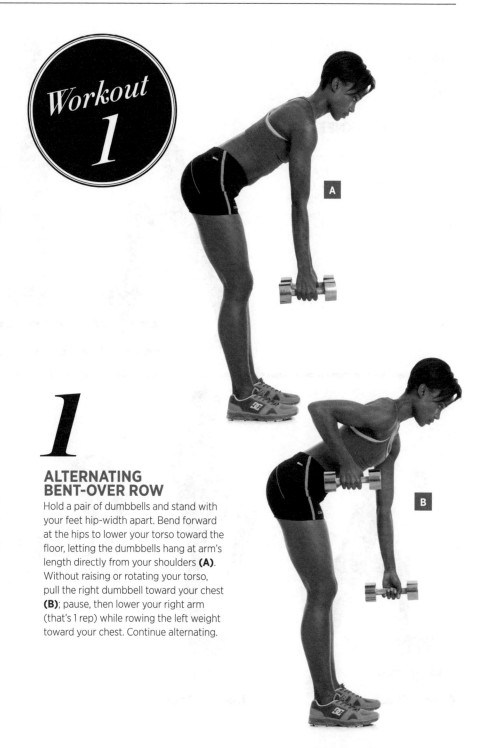

A

B

1

ALTERNATING BENT-OVER ROW

Hold a pair of dumbbells and stand with your feet hip-width apart. Bend forward at the hips to lower your torso toward the floor, letting the dumbbells hang at arm's length directly from your shoulders **(A)**. Without raising or rotating your torso, pull the right dumbbell toward your chest **(B)**; pause, then lower your right arm (that's 1 rep) while rowing the left weight toward your chest. Continue alternating.

2

STEP UP WITH KNEE DRIVE (LEFT)

Stand in front of a step or bench and place your left foot on top of it **(A)**. Push down through your left heel, pressing your body straight up onto the bench while driving your right knee up **(B)**. Reverse the movement to return to the start. That's 1 rep.

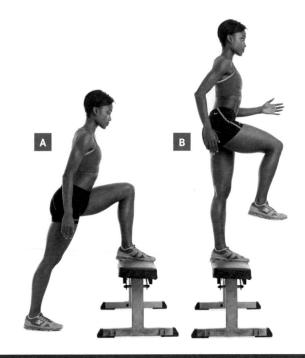

3

STEP UP WITH KNEE DRIVE (RIGHT)

Repeat this exercise using the opposite leg.

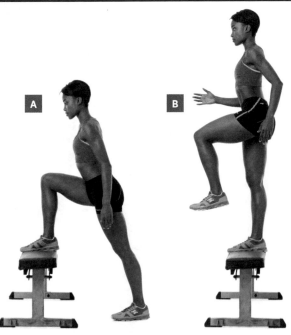

4

PRESS-UP

Place your hands shoulder-width apart on the floor and extend your legs behind you **(A)**. Lower your body until your chest nearly touches the floor **(B)**. Pause, then push back to start as quickly as possible. That's 1 rep.

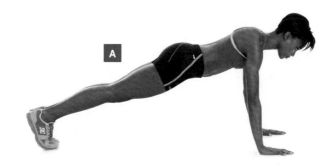

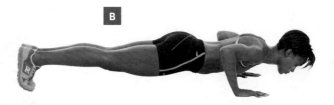

5

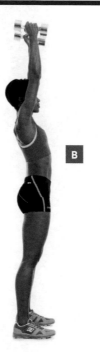

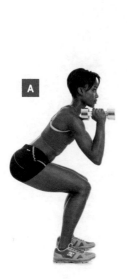

DUMBBELL SQUAT AND OVERHEAD PRESS

Hold a pair of dumbbells at shoulder height and stand with your feet hip-width apart, then sit your hips back and lower into a squat **(A)**. Push through your heels to stand, pressing the dumbbells overhead **(B)**. Lower the weights to the starting position. That's 1 rep.

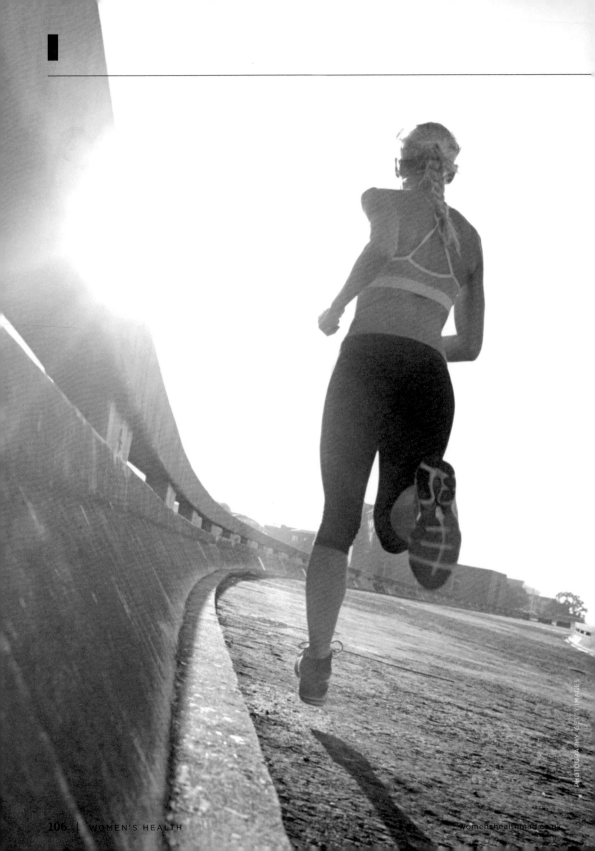

Workout 2

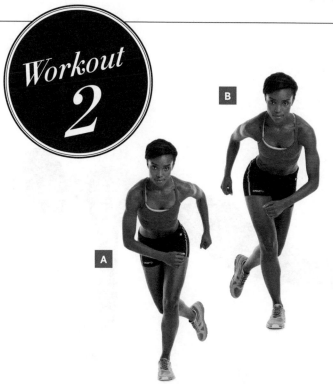

1

SKATER HOPS

Stand on your left foot with your left knee slightly bent and your right foot slightly off the floor **(A)**. Jump to the right and land on your right foot, bringing your left foot **(B)**. That's 1 rep. Jump to the left and continue alternating as quickly as possible.

2

MARCHING GLUTE BRIDGE

Lie on your back with your knees bent, feet flat on the floor. Rest your arms on the floor, palms up. Raise your hips so your body forms a straight line from shoulders to knees **(A)**. Brace your abs and lift your right knee toward your chest **(B)**. Hold for 2 seconds, then lower your right foot. Repeat with the other leg. That's 1 rep.

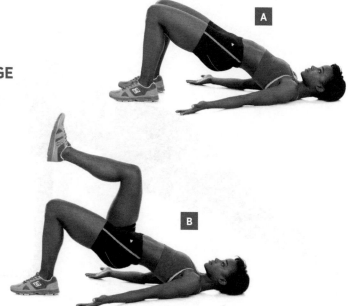

3

ROTATING T EXTENSION

Start in a press-up position **(A)**. Keeping your arms straight and your core engaged, shift your weight onto your left arm, rotate your torso to the right, and raise your right arm toward the ceiling so that your body forms a 'T' **(B)**. Hold for 3 seconds, then return to start and repeat on the other side. That's 1 rep.

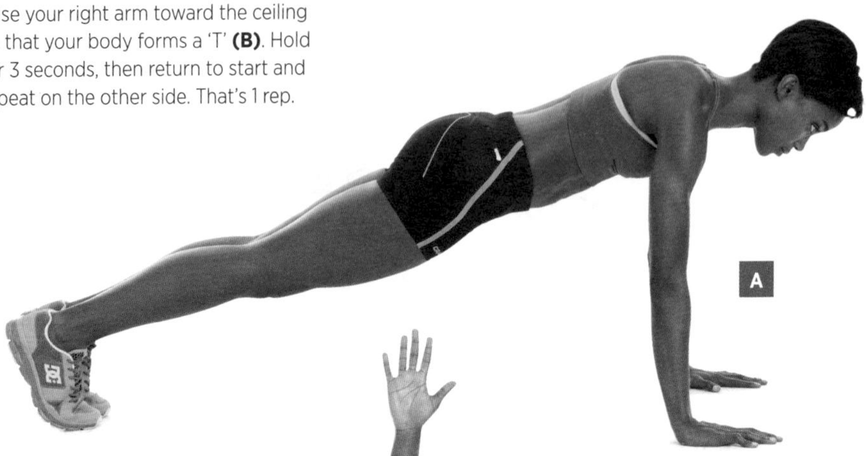

A

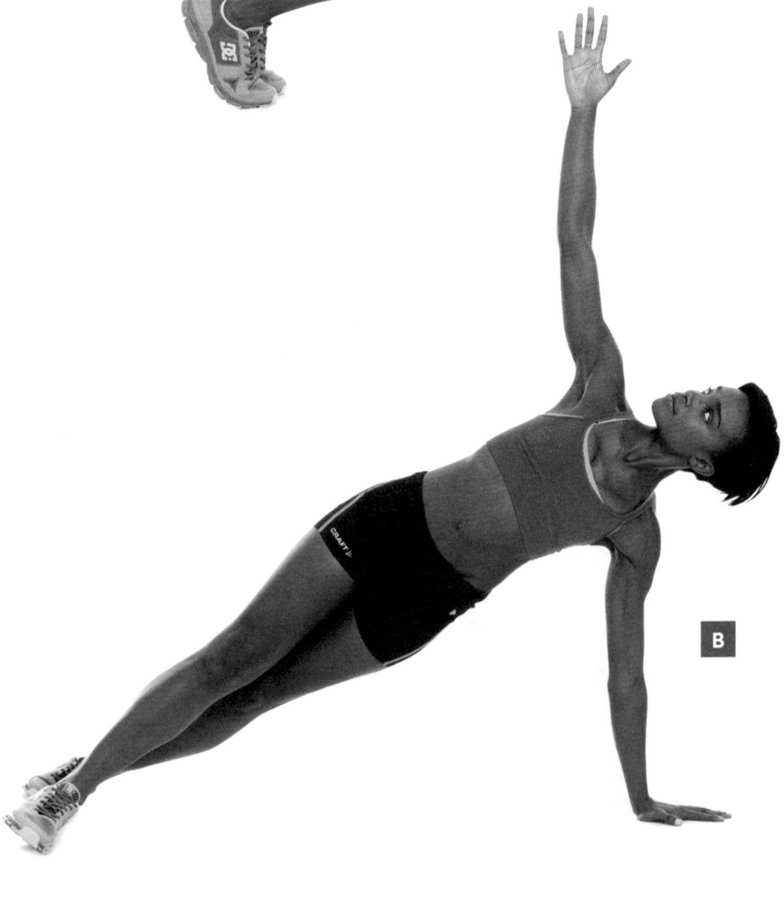

B

4

INVERTED SHOULDER PRESS

Start in a press-up position, hands slightly wider than shoulder width, then move your feet forward and raise your hips so that your torso is nearly perpendicular to the floor **(A)**. From that position, bend your elbows to lower your body until your head nearly touches the floor **(B)**. Pause, push back to start. That's 1 rep.

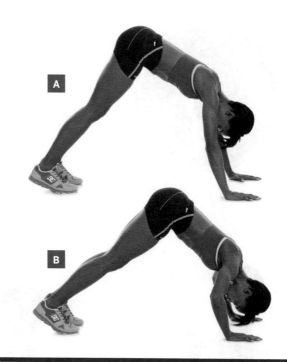

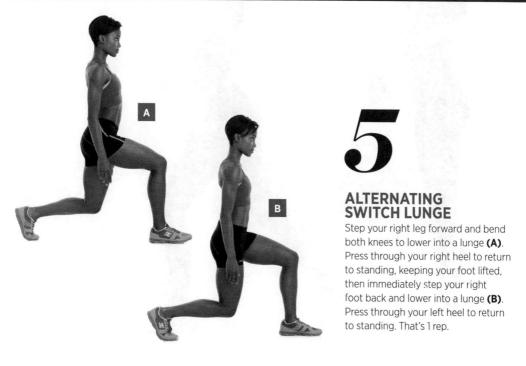

5

ALTERNATING SWITCH LUNGE

Step your right leg forward and bend both knees to lower into a lunge **(A)**. Press through your right heel to return to standing, keeping your foot lifted, then immediately step your right foot back and lower into a lunge **(B)**. Press through your left heel to return to standing. That's 1 rep.

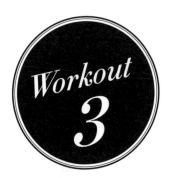

Workout
3

1 DUMBBELL SPLIT JERK

Hold a pair of dumbbells at shoulder height, palms facing each other, feet hip-width apart **(A)**. Dip your knees, then quickly press the dumbbells directly overhead as you jump your legs apart so that you land in a staggered stance, one foot in front of the other **(B)**. Step or jump back to start, lowering the weights back to your shoulders. That's 1 rep.

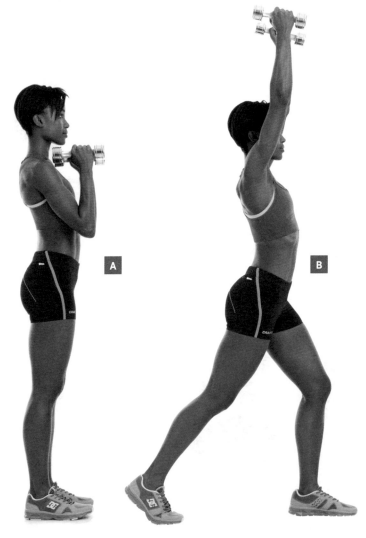

A

B

2

PRESS-UP POSITION ROW

Get into a press-up position with your hands resting on dumbbells, feet slightly more than hip-width apart **(A)**. Pull one weight toward the side of your chest **(B)**. Lower and repeat on the other side. That's 1 rep.

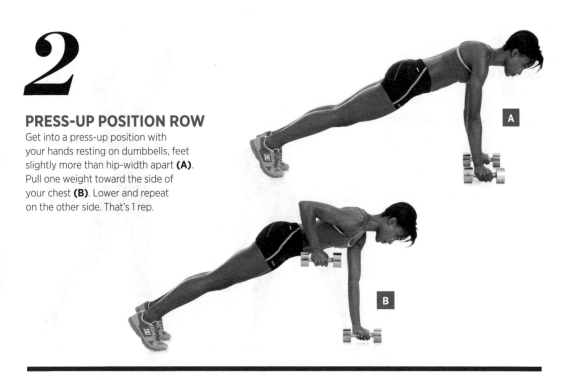

3

ALTERNATING LATERAL LUNGE

Holding a pair of dumbbells at your sides **(A)**, step to the left and bend your right knee to lower into a side lunge. Lower the dumbbells toward your right foot **(B)**. Press through your right heel to return to start. That's 1 rep. Repeat on the other side and continue alternating.

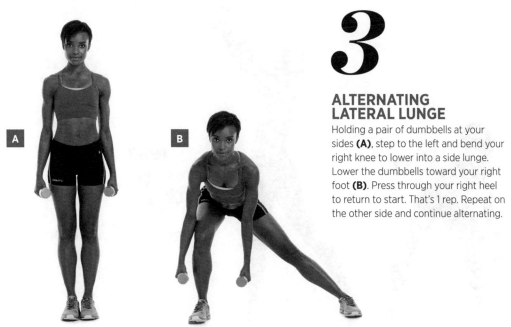

4

REVERSE WOODCHOP

Grab a dumbbell with both hands and stand with your feet wider than hip width, bend your knees, and lower the weight to the side of your left thigh **(A)**. In one motion, press through your heels to stand, and raise the weight over your right shoulder, arms straight and core tight **(B)**. Reverse the movement to return to start. That's 1 rep.

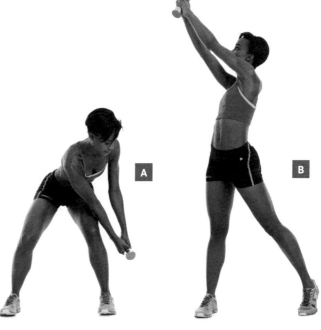

5

REVERSE WOODCHOP

Repeat the above exercise, this time starting with the weight outside your right thigh, and raising it over your left shoulder.

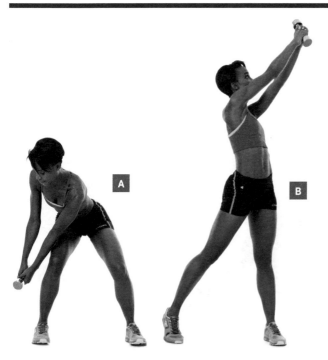

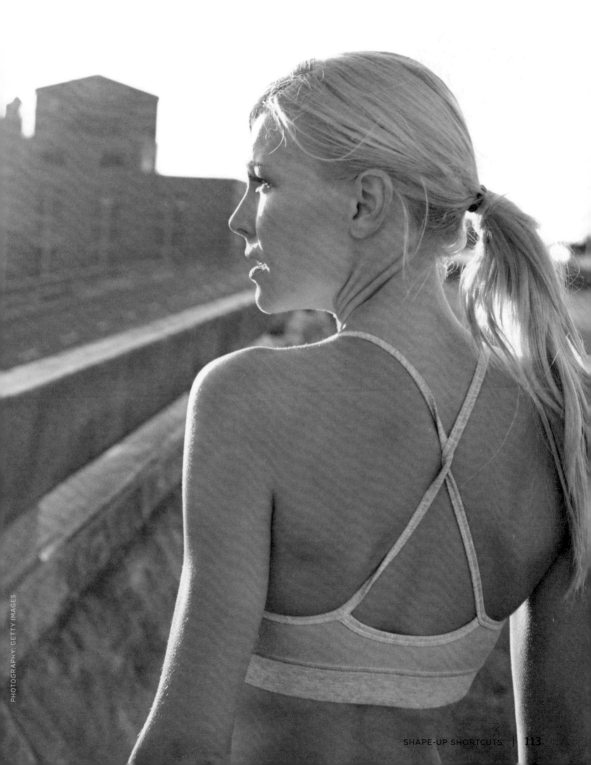

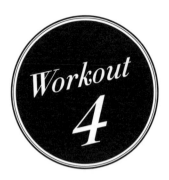

Workout **4**

1

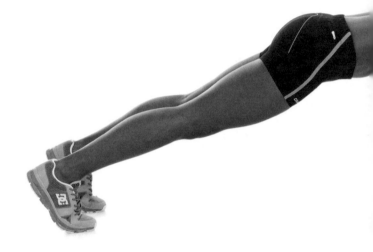

CROSS-BODY MOUNTAIN CLIMBER

Start in a press-up position, core and glutes engaged **(A)**. Keeping your back flat and hips level, bend your right knee toward your left shoulder **(B)**. Return to the start and repeat with your left leg. That's 1 rep.

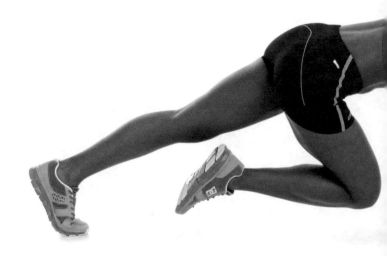

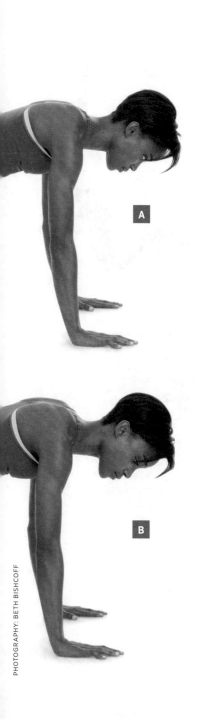

2

STRAIGHT-LEG DUMBBELL DEADLIFT

Hold a pair of dumbbells in front of your thighs, feet hip-width apart **(A)**. Push your hips back and hinge forward to lower your torso until it's almost parallel to the floor, keeping the weights close to your body **(B)**. Return to standing, still keeping the weights close to your body (as if you're shaving your legs with the dumbbells). That's 1 rep. Squeeze your glutes and push your hips forward as you stand. Your hips should initiate the movement, not your chest, to avoid relying on your lower back.

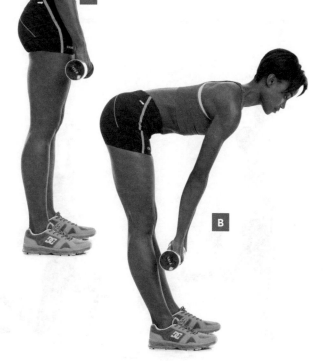

PHOTOGRAPHY: BETH BISHCOFF

3

OVERHEAD DUMBBELL SPLIT SQUAT (RIGHT LEG)

Grab a pair of dumbbells and stand about 2 feet in front of a step or bench; bend your left knee to place the top of your foot on it and raise the weights overhead, arms straight and core tight **(A)**. Bend your knees to lower your body toward the ground **(B)**. Push through your right heel to stand. That's 1 rep.

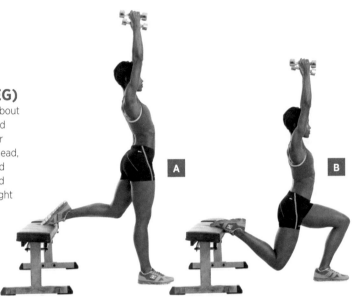

4

OVERHEAD DUMBBELL SPLIT SQUAT (LEFT LEG)

Repeat the above exercise, starting with your right foot on the bench **(A)**. Your hips should stay directly under your body throughout. Think 'drop down' not 'lunge forward.' Holding the weights overhead increases the demand on your core **(B)**. If your form falters, bend your elbows to bring the weights to shoulder height and continue.

SIDE-TO-SIDE JUMPS

Stand with your arms at your sides, feet together **(A)**. Jump to the left with both feet together (imagine you're jumping over a 5-inch cone) **(B)**, landing softly on the balls of your feet; that's 1 rep. Immediately jump to the right, and continue going back and forth as quickly as possible.

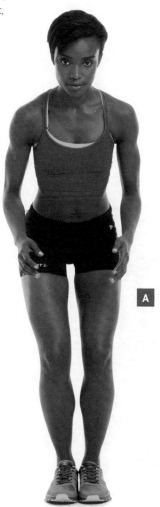

A

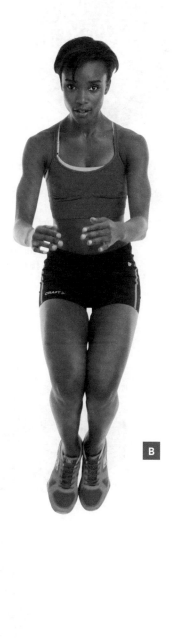

B

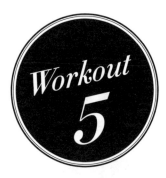

Workout
5

1 BENT-KNEE DEADLIFT

Set a pair of dumbbells on the floor in front of you. Keeping your chest lifted, sit back and bend your knees to squat down and grab the dumbbells with an overhand grip **(A)**. Press through your heels to stand, squeezing your glutes and pushing your hips forward **(B)**. Slowly lower the dumbbells to the floor. That's 1 rep.

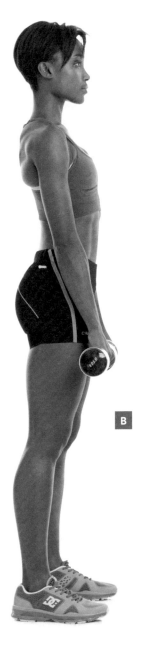

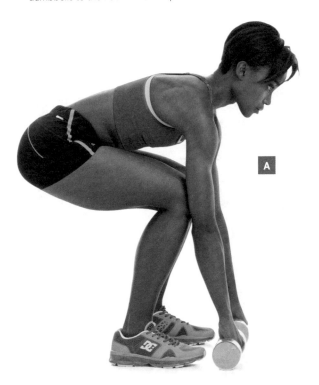

A

B

2

SINGLE-ARM ROTATIONAL ROW (RIGHT ARM)

Stand with your left foot about 2 feet in front of your right, holding a dumbbell in your right hand, palm facing your body. Bend your knees and hinge forward to lower your torso toward the floor, the weight hanging straight from your shoulder **(A)**. Brace your core and pull the dumbbell toward the right side of your chest, rotating your torso to the right **(B)**. Pause, then lower back to start. That's 1 rep.

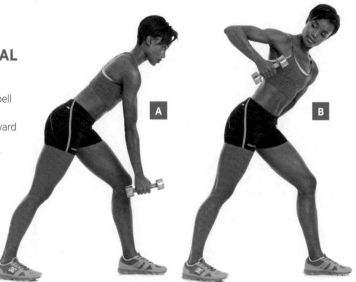

3

SINGLE-ARM ROTATIONAL ROW (LEFT ARM)

Repeat the same exercise, this time with the weight in your left hand and your right foot in front of your left.

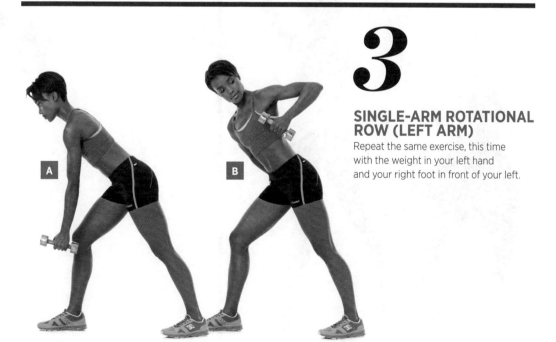

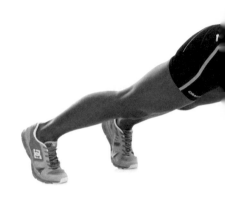

4

GOBLET SQUAT WITH ROTATION AND PRESS

Stand with your feet about hip-width apart and hold a dumbbell vertically in front of your chest, with both hands cupping the dumbbell head **(A)**. Bend your knees and push your hips back to lower your body until your thighs are parallel to the ground. In one motion, stand up and rotate your feet and torso to the left as you press the weight over your left shoulder **(B)**. Reverse the movement to return to start and repeat to the other side. That's 1 rep. Continue alternating.

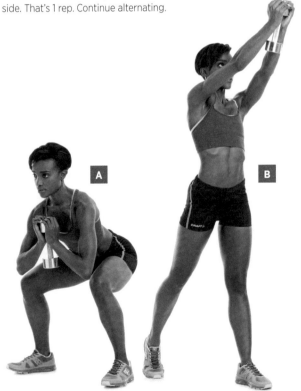

A

B

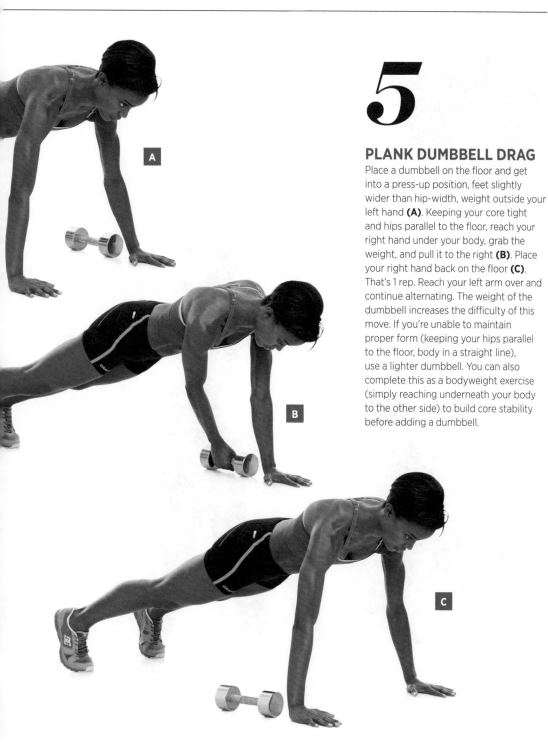

5

PLANK DUMBBELL DRAG

Place a dumbbell on the floor and get into a press-up position, feet slightly wider than hip-width, weight outside your left hand **(A)**. Keeping your core tight and hips parallel to the floor, reach your right hand under your body, grab the weight, and pull it to the right **(B)**. Place your right hand back on the floor **(C)**. That's 1 rep. Reach your left arm over and continue alternating. The weight of the dumbbell increases the difficulty of this move. If you're unable to maintain proper form (keeping your hips parallel to the floor, body in a straight line), use a lighter dumbbell. You can also complete this as a bodyweight exercise (simply reaching underneath your body to the other side) to build core stability before adding a dumbbell.

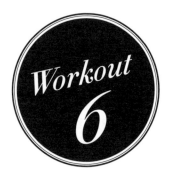

Workout 6

1

SUMO SQUAT WITH LATERAL RAISE

Grab a pair of dumbbells and stand with your feet wider than shoulder-width apart, toes turned out. Sit your hips back and bend your knees to lower into a squat, arms straight and dumbbells between your knees, palms facing each other **(A)**. In one motion, press through your heels to stand and raise both dumbbells to shoulder height **(B)**. Slowly reverse the movement and immediately lower into another rep.

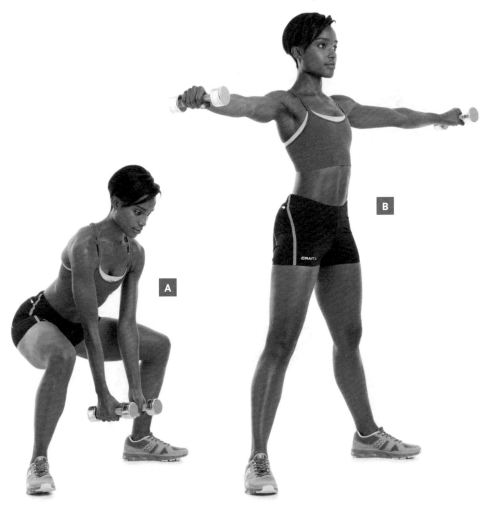

2

DUMBBELL CHEST PRESS

Grab a pair of dumbbells and position your upper back on a bench with your knees bent, feet flat on the floor; raise your hips to form a straight line from shoulders to knees, and press the dumbbells over your chest, arms straight and palms facing away from you **(A)**. Lower your arms until the weights are even with your chest **(B)**. Press back to the starting position. That's 1 rep.

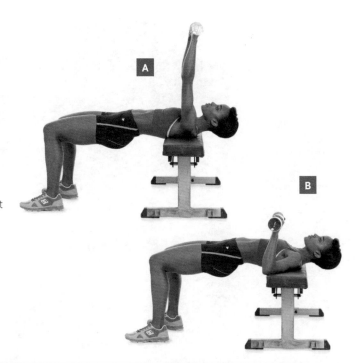

3

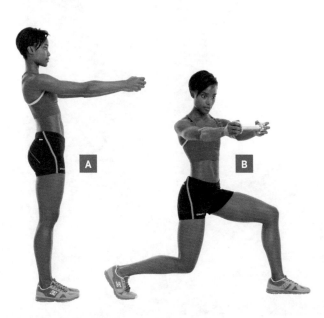

DUMBBELL LUNGE WITH ROTATION

Grab a dumbbell with both hands and raise it to shoulder height in front of you, arms straight and feet hip-width apart **(A)**. Keeping your core tight and your chest up, step forward with your left foot and lower your body until your front thigh is nearly parallel to the floor, rotating your shoulders and torso to the right **(B)**. Rotate back to the centre as you press through your right heel to return to the standing position. That's 1 rep. Repeat on the other side and continue alternating.

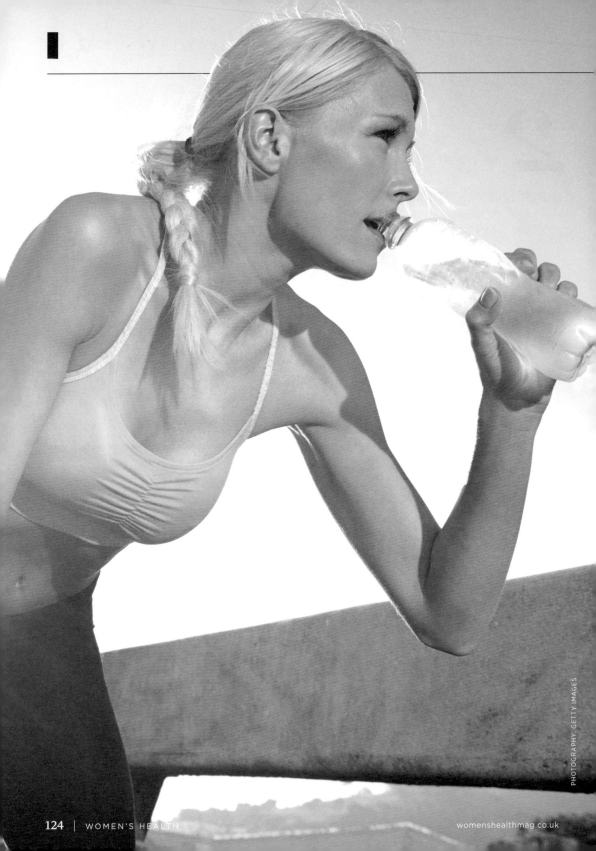

4

PLANK WALK-UP

Position your forearms on the ground, elbows directly under your shoulders, and extend your legs behind you **(A)**. Place your right hand flat on the floor **(B)**, and then your left hand, straightening your arms to press your body into a press-up position **(C)**. Reverse the movement, lowering onto your right forearm and then your left, to return to the start. That's 1 rep. Repeat, leading with your left hand, and continue alternating.

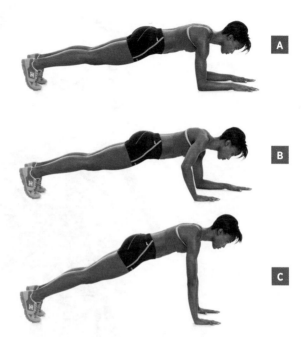

5

LOW-BOX LATERAL SHUFFLE

Stand to the right of a low box or step and place your left foot on it; bend your knees slightly and keep your chest up **(A)**. Push off your left foot and jump over the box to your left, landing with your right foot on the box and your left foot on the floor, knees bent **(B)**. Quickly return to start. That's 1 rep.

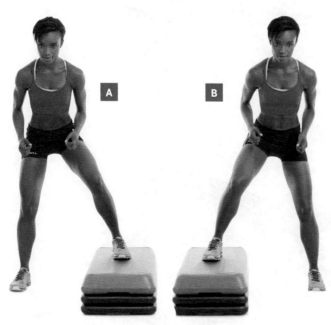

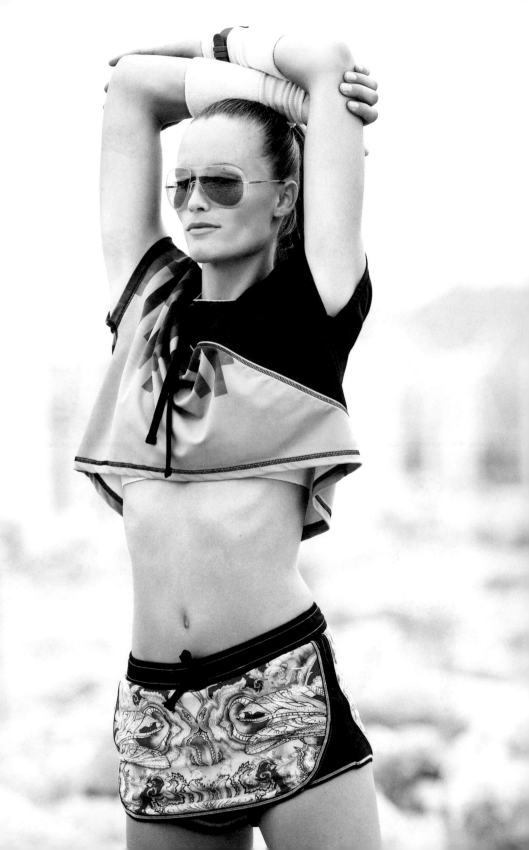

KEEP IT SIMPLE

Slim down faster, with less equipment

These innovative routines are scientifically designed to give you the most effective workout in under 30 minutes, using just one piece of equipment (or none!). They're all about simplicity: you'll focus on essentials in your sweat-session to get the most out of every rep, every set, every minute. So, no stumbling from one piece of equipment to the next – or worse, queuing to work out during gym rush hour. Whether you're at the gym or exercising at home, there's a routine that will work for you.

THE
GREATEST
BODYWEIGHT
WORKOUT
No gym, no equipment –
just lean and toned muscle
EVER

Y ou don't need a gym membership to sculpt a great body. You don't even need equipment. Think about the classic pull-up – for many women, it's hideously hard, and there are no weights involved. When you do a pull-up, your body is in a position that forces your back and arms to lift your entire body weight; the laws of motion and leverage work against you. So, physics turns your body into a super-efficient resistance machine.

The problem is, over time your body adapts and basic body weight exercises – even dreaded chin-ups – get easier. Increasing your reps can offset the plateau, but only to an extent.

This workout has three distinct phases that increase in difficulty, so you don't get stuck at a plateau. During each phase, you'll move quickly through four compound sets. Like the superset, compound sets are a time-saver because you progress from one move to the next with no rest.

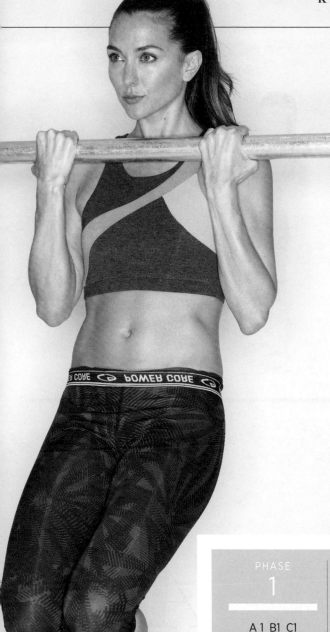

Unlike supersets, which work opposing muscle groups, compound sets work the same muscle group back to back. Take the first two moves: a bodyweight squat followed by an isometric wall squat. This helps recruit even more muscle fibres and creates greater strength gains – all without adding external resistance.

Here's how you do it

Start with Workout 1. Refer to the directions for Phase 1 in the box below, and complete the required reps for A1 and A2 without rest. Move on to B1 and B2 and repeat, and continue until you've finished all the exercises. A full round of all four compound sets makes one circuit. Rest for 60 seconds, then repeat for two to four total circuits.

There are three ways to make this workout more challenging First, you could increase the volume by moving through the three phases using the same workout: the reps and duration increase. You can also increase the exercise difficulty by going from Workout 1, to Workout 2, to Workout 3 but keeping the phase the same. Finally, you can change both factors – volume and exercise difficulty – at the same time. Start in Phase 1 with Workout 1, then move to Phase 2 with Workout 2, and finally Phase 3 with Workout 3.

PHASE 1	PHASE 2	PHASE 3
A 1 B1 C1	A 1 B1 C1	A 1 B1 C1
10 REPS	**15 REPS**	**20 REPS**
A2 B2 C2 D1 D2	A2 B2 C2 D1 D2	A2 B2 C2 D1 D2
30 seconds	**40 seconds**	**60 seconds**
(or 15 each side)	(or 20 each side)	(or 30 each side)

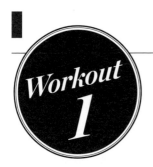

A1

BODYWEIGHT SQUAT

Stand with your feet slightly wider than hip-width apart, and raise your arms straight in front of you at shoulder height **(A)**. Keeping your arms straight and your chest lifted, sit your hips back and bend your knees to lower your body until your thighs are parallel to the ground **(B)**. Pause, then press through your heels to return to standing. That's 1 rep.

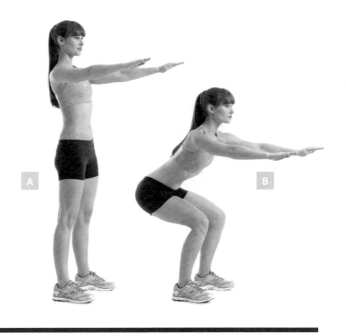

A

B

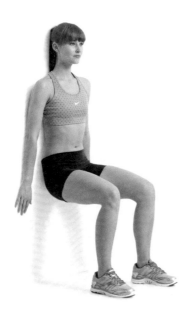

A2

ISOMETRIC WALL SQUAT

Stand with your back against a wall, your feet about 2 feet in front of you, hip-width apart. Bend your knees to lower your body until your knees are bent at 90 degrees. Hold.

B1

MODIFIED WIDE-GRIP PRESS-UP

Start in a press-up position with your hands wider than shoulder-width apart on the floor, then place your knees on the ground, so your body forms a straight line from shoulders to knees **(A)**. Bend your elbows to lower your body toward the floor in a straight line **(B)**. Press back up to the start. That's 1 rep.

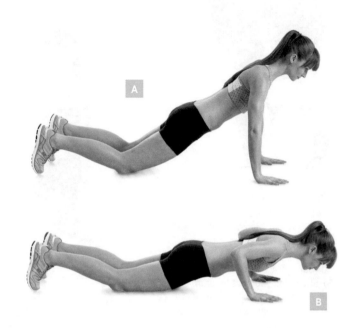

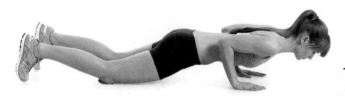

B2

NARROW-GRIP MODIFIED ISOMETRIC PRESS-UP

Start in a press-up position with your hands closer than shoulder-width apart on the floor, then place your knees on the ground, so your body forms a straight line from shoulders to knees. Bend your elbows to lower your body until your elbows form 90-degree angles. Hold.

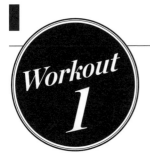
C1

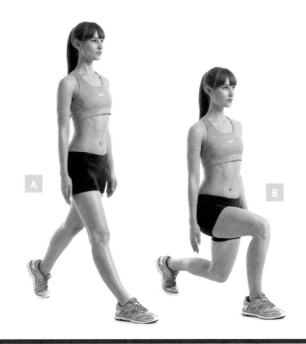

A

B

SPLIT SQUAT

Stand with your legs staggered, your right foot about 2 feet in front of your left **(A)**. Bend your knees to lower your body until your right thigh is parallel and your shin is perpendicular to the floor **(B)**. Straighten your legs to return to the start. That's 1 rep. Complete all reps on that leg, then switch sides and repeat.

C2

GLUTE BRIDGE

Lie face up on the floor with your knees bent, feet flat on the floor, and your arms to your sides, palms facing up. Press through your heels and raise your hips off the ground, so your body forms a straight line from shoulders to knees. Hold.

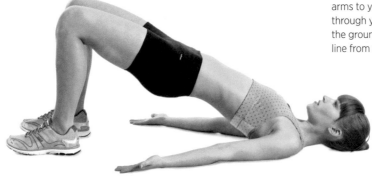

D1

PLANK

Place your forearms on the ground with your elbows directly under your shoulders, and extend your legs so that your body forms a straight line from head to heels. Brace your core and hold.

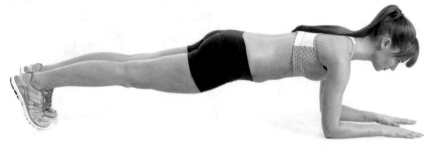

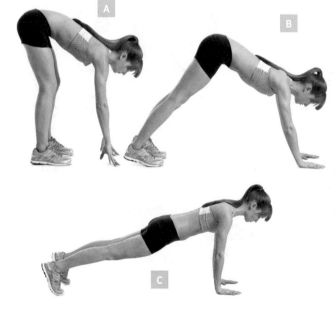

D2

INCHWORM

Stand with your feet hip-width apart, bend over, and touch the floor in front of your feet with both hands **(A)**. Keeping your legs straight and core tight, walk your hands forward as far as you can without letting your hips drop **(B, C)**. Pause, then slowly walk your feet toward your hands. That's 1 rep.

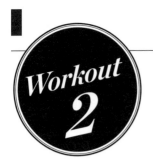
A1

ALTERNATING LATERAL LUNGE

Stand with your feet hip-width apart, arms raised to shoulder height **(A)**. Keeping your arms raised and your chest lifted, step out to the left with your left leg; bend your knee and sit back to lower into a side lunge **(B)**. Return to standing. That's 1 rep; repeat on the other side and continue alternating.

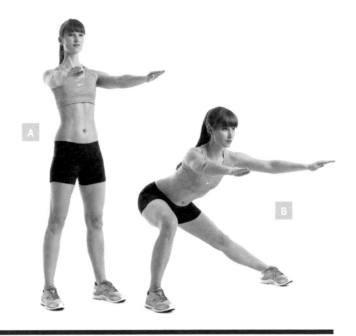

A2

ALTERNATING LEG ISOMETRIC WALL SQUAT

Stand with your back against a wall, your feet about 2 feet in front of you, hip-width apart. Bend your knees to lower your body until your knees are bent at 90 degrees **(A)**. Extend your right leg out in front of you, shin parallel to the floor **(B)**. Hold for 1 or 2 seconds, then switch sides and repeat. Continue alternating.

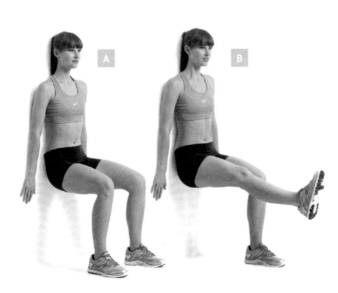

B1

WIDE-GRIP PRESS-UP

Place your hands on the floor, wider than shoulder-width apart, and extend your feet behind you into a press-up position, so your body forms a straight line from head to heels **(A)**. Bend your elbows to lower your body toward the floor **(B)**. Press back up to the start. That's 1 rep.

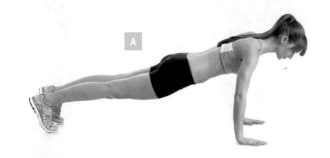

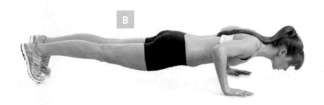

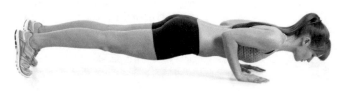

B2

NARROW-GRIP ISOMETRIC PUSHUP

Place your hands on the floor closer than shoulder-width apart, and extend your feet behind you into a press-up position, so your body forms a straight line from head to heels. Keeping your core tight, bend your elbows to lower your body in a straight line until your elbows form 90-degree angles. Hold.

C1

ALTERNATING REVERSE LUNGE

Stand with your feet hip-width apart, arms at your sides **(A)**. Step back with your left leg and lower your body until your right knee is bent at 90 degrees **(B)**. Push back up to the start. That's 1 rep. Complete all reps on that leg, then switch sides and repeat.

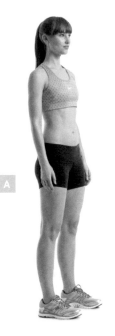
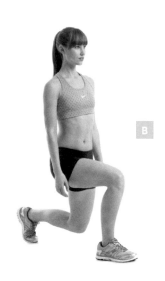

C2

MARCHING GLUTE BRIDGE

Lie face up on the floor with your knees bent, feet flat on the floor, and your arms to your sides, palms facing up. Press through your heels and raise your hips off the ground so your body forms a straight line from shoulders to knees **(A)**. From this position, raise your right foot off the ground, knee bent at 90 degrees, until your shin is parallel to the floor **(B)**. Hold for 2 or 3 seconds, then lower your right foot and repeat with the left foot. Continue alternating.

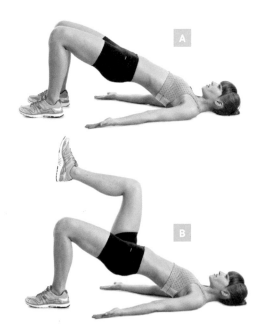

D1

SIDE PLANK

Lie on your left side and place your forearm on the ground with your elbow directly under your shoulder, your legs straight and stacked. Lift your hips so your body forms a straight line from head to heels. Hold, then switch sides and repeat.

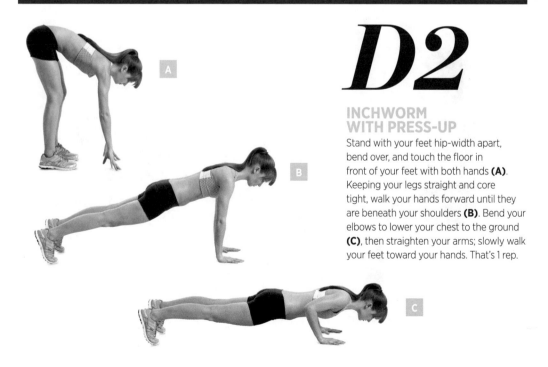

D2

INCHWORM WITH PRESS-UP

Stand with your feet hip-width apart, bend over, and touch the floor in front of your feet with both hands **(A)**. Keeping your legs straight and core tight, walk your hands forward until they are beneath your shoulders **(B)**. Bend your elbows to lower your chest to the ground **(C)**, then straighten your arms; slowly walk your feet toward your hands. That's 1 rep.

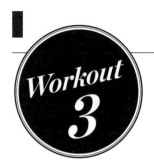

A1

SINGLE-LEG BODYWEIGHT SQUAT

Stand with your feet hip-width apart, arms raised to shoulder height **(A)**, and raise your left foot off the ground. Sit your hips back and bend your right knee to lower your body, keeping your left leg off the ground **(B)**. Press through your heel to return to standing. Complete all reps on that leg, then switch sides and repeat.

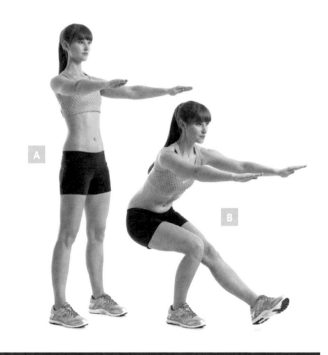

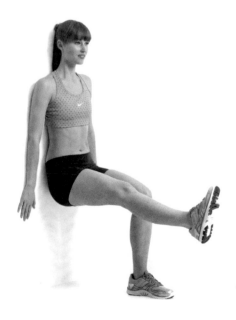

A2

SINGLE-LEG ISOMETRIC WALL SQUAT

Stand with your back against a wall, your feet about 2 feet in front of you, hip-width apart. Bend your knees to lower your body until your knees are bent at 90 degrees. Extend your right leg out in front of you, shin parallel to the floor. Hold for 1 or 2 seconds, then switch sides and repeat. Continue alternating.

B1

SINGLE-LEG WIDE-GRIP PRESS-UP

Place your hands on the floor wider than shoulder-width apart, and extend your feet behind you into a press-up position, so your body forms a straight line from head to heels. Raise your left leg **(A)**, then bend your elbows to lower your body toward the floor in a straight line **(B)**. Press back up to the start and lower your leg. That's 1 rep. Repeat on the other side and continue alternating.

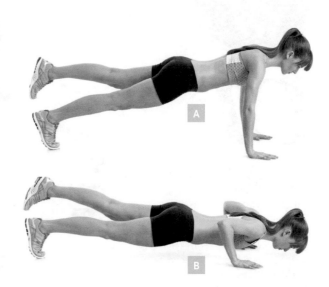

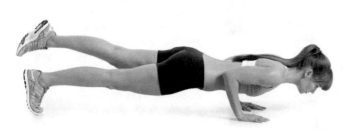

B2

SINGLE-LEG NARROW-GRIP PRESS-UP

Place your hands on the floor closer than shoulder-width apart, and extend your feet behind you into a press-up position, so your body forms a straight line from head to heels. Raise your left leg, then bend your elbows to lower your body until your elbows form 90-degree angles. Hold.

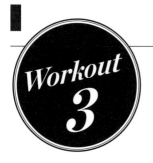

C1

REAR-FOOT ELEVATED SPLIT SQUAT

Stand 2 feet in front of a step or bench and place the top of your left foot on it **(A)**. Bend your knees to lower into a lunge, until your left knee grazes the floor, keeping your hips directly under your body **(B)**. Push through your right heel to stand. That's 1 rep. Complete all reps with that leg, then switch sides and repeat.

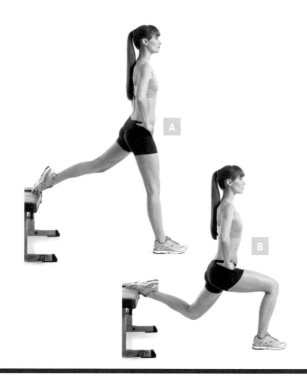

C2

SINGLE-LEG HIP EXTENSION

Lie face up on the floor with your left knee bent and your right leg straight **(A)**. Raise your right leg until it's in line with your left thigh. Push your hips upwards, keeping your right leg elevated, until your body forms a straight line from shoulders to right ankle **(B)**. Pause, then slowly lower your body and leg back to the start. That's 1 rep. Complete all the reps with that leg, then switch sides and repeat.

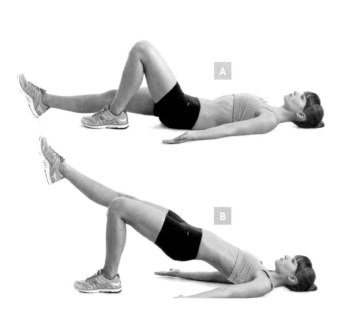

D1

ROLLING PLANK

Start in the plank position, with your forearms on the ground and your legs extended behind you **(A)**. Rotate your torso to the side, rolling onto your left forearm and stacking your right foot on top of your left in a left-side plank **(B)**. Pause, then return to the start, and repeat on the other side.

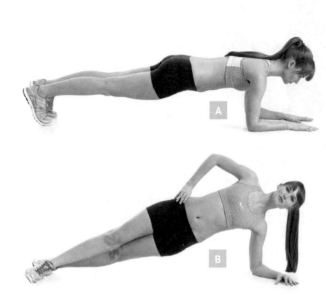

D2

BURPEE

Stand with your feet slightly wider than shoulder-width apart, arms at your sides. Push your hips back, bend your knees, and lower your body into a squat and place both hands on the floor in front of you **(A)**. Jump both feet back into a press-up position **(B)**. Bring your feet back into a low squat and quickly jump up into the air, swinging your arms overhead then moving back to standing position **(C)**. That's 1 rep.

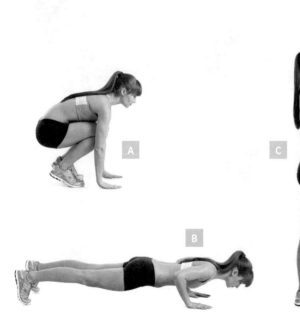

Circuit 1

TONE EVERY INCH

Build a stronger, leaner body from head to toe and burn fat fast with this workout. Starting with Circuit 1, complete the prescribed number of reps for each exercise, moving from one to the next without resting. Repeat for a total of three sets, then rest two minutes. Follow the same pattern to complete three sets of Circuit 2, then continue to Circuit 3 and perform two sets.

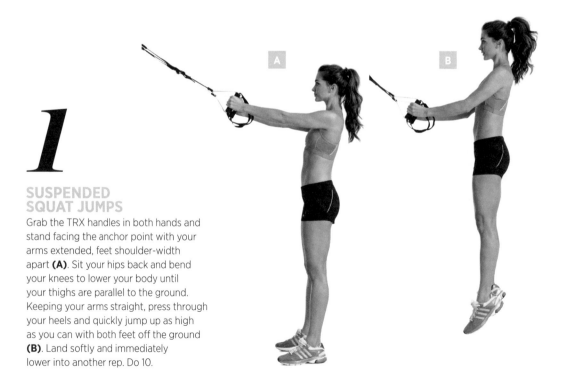

1

SUSPENDED SQUAT JUMPS

Grab the TRX handles in both hands and stand facing the anchor point with your arms extended, feet shoulder-width apart **(A)**. Sit your hips back and bend your knees to lower your body until your thighs are parallel to the ground. Keeping your arms straight, press through your heels and quickly jump up as high as you can with both feet off the ground **(B)**. Land softly and immediately lower into another rep. Do 10.

2

SUSPENDED CHEST PRESS

Stand facing away from the anchor point, feet hip-width apart, and hold the handles in front of you with arms extended at shoulder height, palms facing the floor **(A)**. Walk your feet away from you and lean forward so your body forms a straight line from head to heels. Keeping your core tight, bend your elbows to lower your chest toward the handles **(B)**. Pause, then press back to the start. That's 1 rep. Do 10.

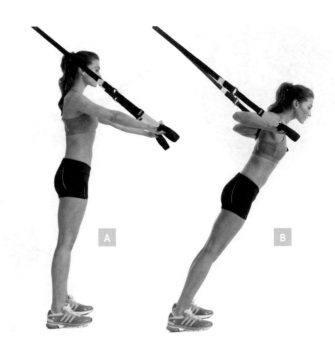

3

SUSPENDED ROW

Grab the TRX handles in both hands and stand facing the anchor point, with feet shoulder-width apart and arms straight in front of you. Lean back and walk your feet forward to the appropriate resistance angle **(A)**. Keeping your shoulders pulled down and back, bend your elbows to pull your chest toward the handles **(B)**. Pause, then return to the start with a slow, controlled movement. That's 1 rep. Do 10.

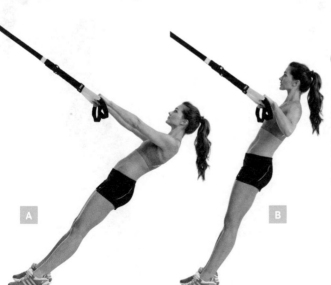

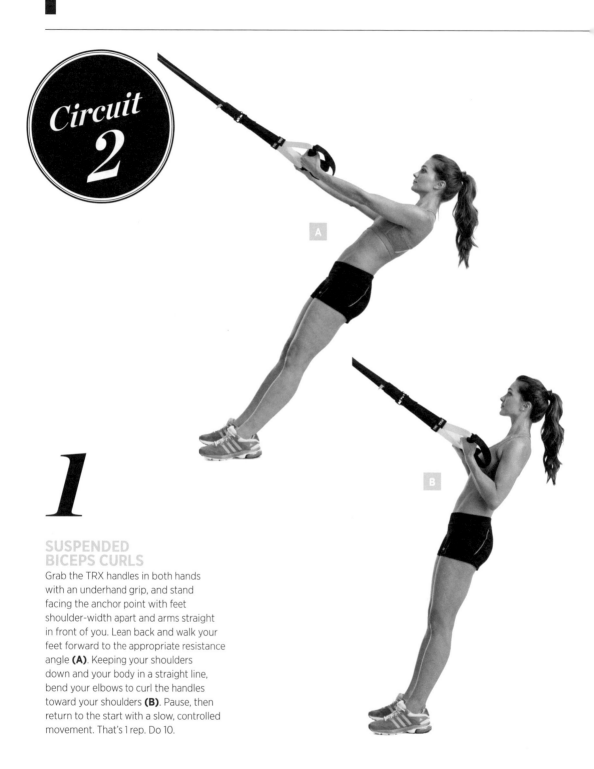

1

SUSPENDED BICEPS CURLS

Grab the TRX handles in both hands with an underhand grip, and stand facing the anchor point with feet shoulder-width apart and arms straight in front of you. Lean back and walk your feet forward to the appropriate resistance angle **(A)**. Keeping your shoulders down and your body in a straight line, bend your elbows to curl the handles toward your shoulders **(B)**. Pause, then return to the start with a slow, controlled movement. That's 1 rep. Do 10.

2

SUSPENDED OVERHEAD TRICEPS EXTENSIONS

Stand facing away from the anchor point, feet hip-width apart, and hold the handles with your palms facing down and your arms extended **(A)**. Pressing your body weight into the handles, bend your elbows and lower your body until your hands are behind your head **(B)**. Drive your hands forward and extend your arms to return to the start. That's 1 rep. Do 10.

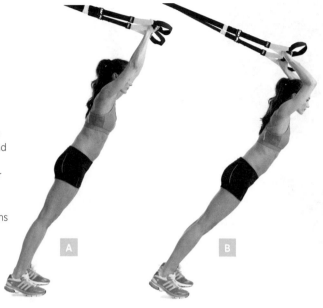

3

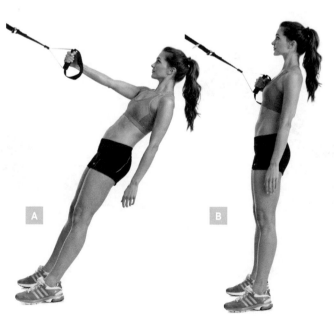

SUSPENDED POWER PULL

Stand facing the anchor point, feet hip-width apart, and hold one handle in your right hand, arm extended at shoulder height. Lean back and walk your feet forward to the appropriate resistance angle **(A)**. Keeping your core tight and your body in a straight line, bend your right elbow to pull your chest toward the handle **(B)**. Pause, then return to the start. That's 1 rep. Do 8, then switch sides and repeat.

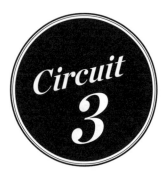

Circuit 3

 1

BURPEE

Stand with your feet about shoulder-width apart **(A)**, then push your hips back and squat down to place your hands on the floor **(B)**. Jump your legs back into a press-up position **(C)**; quickly reverse the movement to return to the start. That's 1 rep. Do 10.

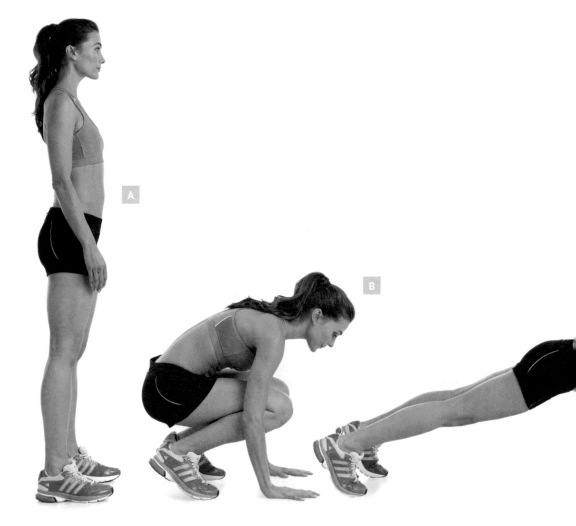

A

B

SKATER JUMP

Cross your left leg behind your right and lower into a half-squat, your right arm out to the side, left arm across your hips **(A)**. Hop to the left, switching your legs and arms **(B)**. That's 1 rep. Keep hopping quickly from side to side. Do 30.

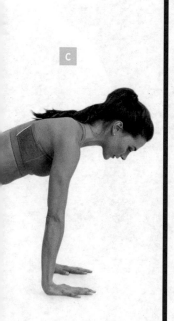

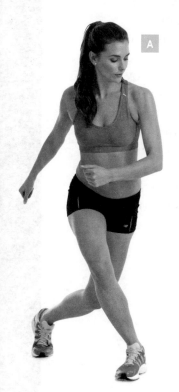

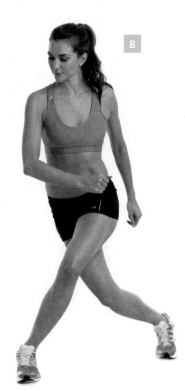

ONE DUMBBELL, ONE HOT BODY

This routine will incinerate fat and tighten your body in record time. Starting with the first exercise, perform the required reps, then rest for 30 seconds before continuing to the next move. You can rest up to a minute – or make things harder by reducing your rest break, or dropping it. Repeat until you've finished the entire circuit, and rest for two minutes. That's one set. Aim to finish as many sets as you can in the time you have, up to 30 minutes. Beginners, start with two sets and increase your number as your stamina builds.

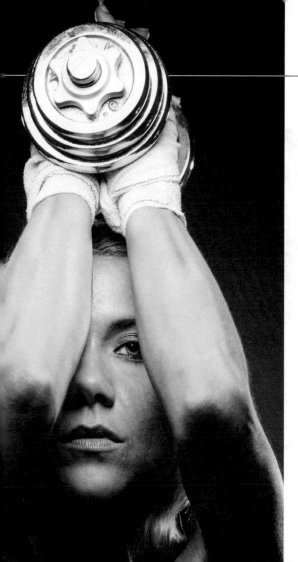

1

NARROW-STANCE GOBLET SQUAT

Stand with your feet shoulder-width apart and hold a dumbbell vertically in front of your chest, both hands cupping the dumbbell head **(A)**. Keeping your chest up and your core tight, sit your hips back and squat as low as you can **(B)**. Press through your heels to return to start. That's 1 rep. Do 15.

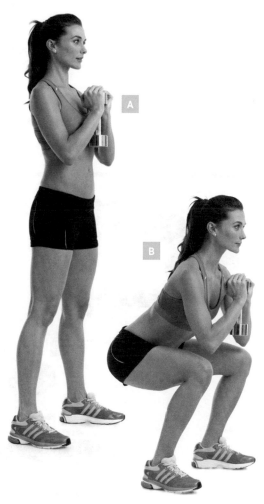

2

GOBLET SPLIT-SQUAT

Stand with your right foot 2 feet in front of your left and hold a dumbbell vertically in front of your chest **(A)**. Bend your knees to lower your body until your right thigh is parallel to the floor **(B)**. Straighten your legs to return to the start. That's 1 rep. Do 6, then switch legs and repeat.

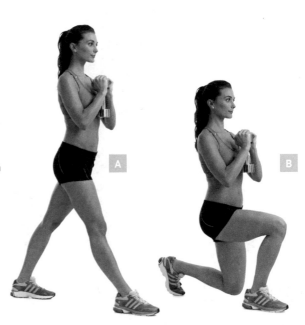

3

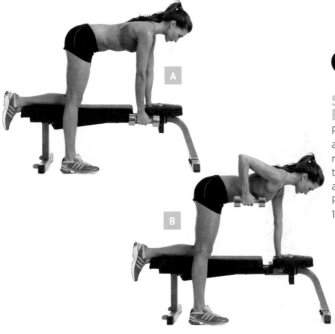

SINGLE-ARM BENT-OVER ROW

Place your left knee and left hand on a bench and hold a dumbbell in your right hand at arm's length, palm facing the bench **(A)**. Slowly bend your elbow and pull the dumbbell to your chest **(B)**. Pause, then lower back to the start. That's 1 rep. Do 10, then repeat on the other side.

4

SINGLE-ARM CHEST PRESS

Lie face up on a bench, holding a dumbbell in your left hand at chest height **(A)**. Press the weight directly over your shoulder **(B)**. Slowly lower back to start. That's 1 rep. Do 10, then switch arms and repeat.

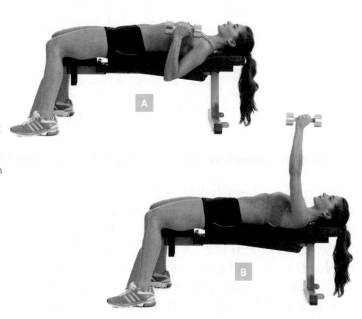

5

DUMBBELL SWING

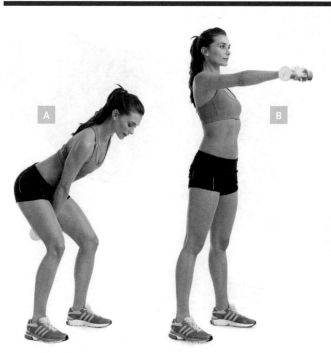

Grab a dumbbell with an overhand grip, feet hip-width apart. Push your hips back, knees slightly bent, and lower your chest to bring the dumbbell between your legs **(A)**. Keeping your core tight, push your hips forward and swing the dumbbell up to shoulder height **(B)**. Reverse the movement, swinging the weight back between your legs. That's 1 rep. Do 15.

THE ULTIMATE KETTLEBELL WORKOUT

If you thought kettlebells were just hyped-up dumbbells, think again. Unlike a dumbbell, a kettlebell's centre of gravity shifts during an exercise, increasing the challenge and building coordination. Researchers found that people who did 20-minute kettlebell workouts torched almost 300 calories – and that's just for starters. When you factor in the calories burned after you exercise as your body repairs its muscle fibres, the total expenditure could increase by up to 50%. Shed fat fast with this metabolism-boosting kettlebell routine Start with Step 1: complete each exercise as instructed, moving from one to the next without rest. Then rest for up to 60 seconds, and repeat for a total of three to five rounds. Then move to Step 2: it'll take 5 to 10 minutes, but it's the secret to dialling up your metabolism after you're finished.

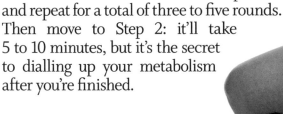

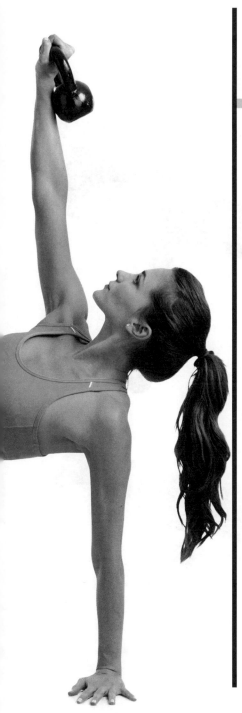

Sculpt sexy muscle

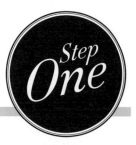

Step **One**

1

KETTLEBELL SUMO DEADLIFT

Stand with your feet about twice shoulder-width apart and your toes pointed out at an angle. Bend at your hips and knees and grab the kettlebell handle with an overhand grip. Your lower back should be slightly arched, and your arms should be straight **(A)**. Without allowing your lower back to round, pull your torso back and up, thrust your hips forward, and stand up with the kettlebell **(B)**. That's 1 rep. Do 12 to 15.

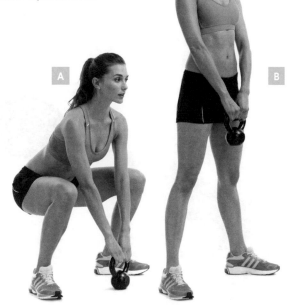

A

B

2 KETTLEBELL PRESS-UP POSITION ROW

Get in a press-up position with your hand on top of a kettlebell **(A)**. Keeping your hips parallel and back flat, bend your elbow to row the weight toward your chest **(B)**. Pause, then return to start. That's 1 rep. Do 8 to 10, then switch sides and repeat.

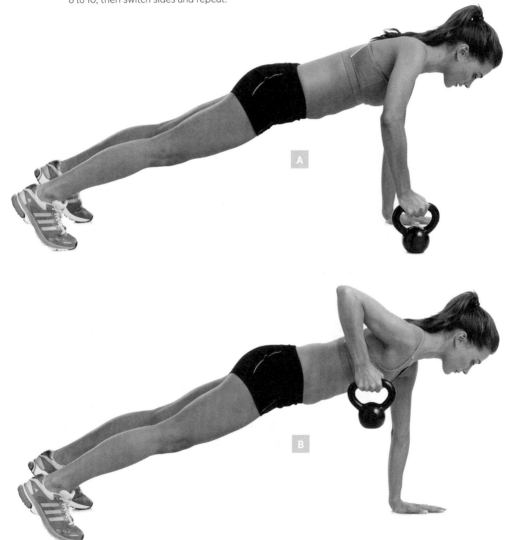

3

KETTLEBELL REVERSE LUNGE

Hold the kettlebell handle in your right hand, so the bell rests on the back of your forearm ('racked' position), hand close to your chest and elbow close to your body **(A)**. Brace your core and step back with your right leg and bend both knees to lower your body until both knees form 90-degree angles **(B)**. Pause, then press through your left heel to return to the start. That's 1 rep. Do 10 to 12, then switch sides and repeat.

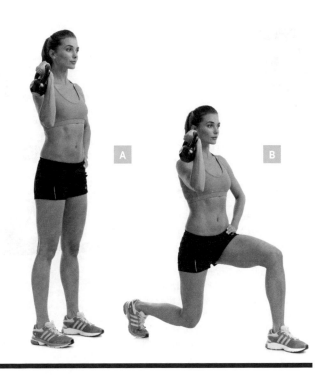

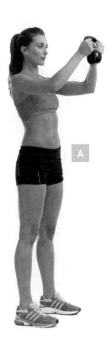

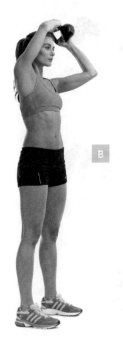

4

KETTLEBELL HALO

Stand with your feet hip-width apart and hold the kettlebell in front of your head, about shoulder height **(A)**. Keeping your core tight and stable, circle the weight counter-clockwise around your head **(B)**. That's 1 rep. Do 12 to 15.

5

KETTLEBELL HALF GET-UP

Lie face up on the floor with your right knee bent, foot flat on the floor, and your left leg extended straight; hold a kettlebell in your right hand, with your arm directly over your shoulder **(A)**. Roll onto your left forearm and punch the ceiling with your right hand to raise your upper body off the ground **(B)**. Straighten your left arm and place your hand on the floor behind you, so that your upper body forms a T; then press into your right heel and raise your hips until they're in line with your knee, raising the weight toward the ceiling **(C)**. Pause, then reverse the movement to return to the starting position. That's 1 rep. Do 8 to 10, then switch sides and repeat.

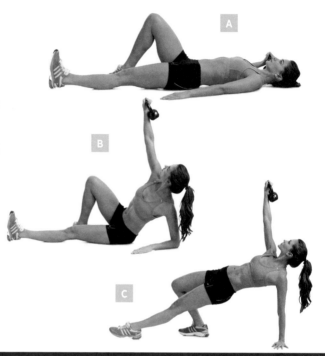

6

YOGA PRESS-UP

Place your hands on the ground directly under your shoulders and extend your legs behind you into a press-up position, with your body forming a straight line **(A)**. Bend your elbows to lower your chest toward the ground **(B)**; straighten your arms and as you return to the start, raise your hips up in the air while driving your heels into the ground (downward-facing dog position) **(C)**. Reset to the starting position. That's 1 rep.

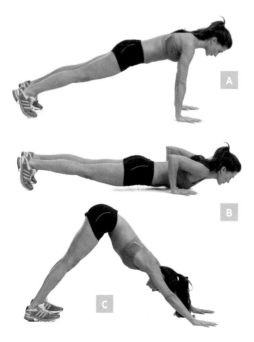

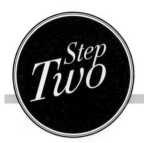

Step Two

Fire up your fat-burners

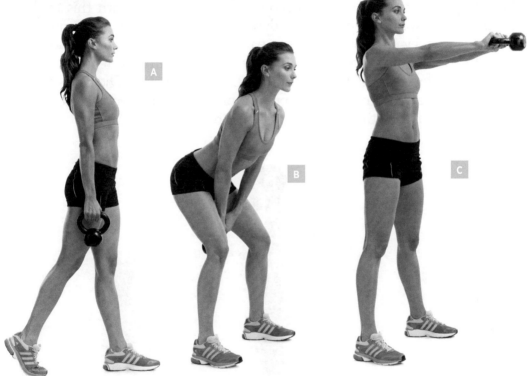

A

B

C

1 SINGLE-ARM FARMER'S WALK SHUTTLE WITH KETTLEBELL SWINGS

Set up two markers 25-30 yards apart. Hold a kettlebell at your right side; walk from one marker to the other, keeping your chest upright **(A)**. Once you reach the other end, position your feet about hip-width apart and hold the kettlebell in front of you with both hands. Push your hips back, slightly bend your knees and lower your chest to bring the weight between your legs **(B)**. Quickly push your hips forward and swing the weight to chest height **(C)**. Immediately bring the weight between your legs. That's 1 rep. Do 10. Hold the kettlebell in your left hand and walk back to the first marker. Perform another 10 swings. That's one round. Rest 30 to 60 seconds. Repeat for two to four rounds.

STEP UP
YOUR RESULTS

Crank up your calorie-burn and score a fierce physique with this explosive 15-minute workout. The innovative, dynamic exercises boost agility and speed, and because they probably don't form part of your everyday routine, you'll stay more focused on the movements. Using a traditional aerobics step (or a 10-15cm low box), perform the following circuit as instructed below. The key is to move quickly while always maintaining proper form. Challenge yourself to squeeze out an extra rep each time you complete this routine.

1

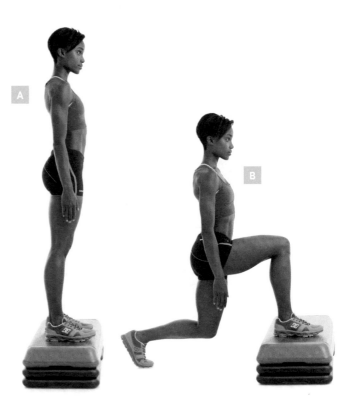

ALTERNATING ELEVATED REVERSE LUNGE

Stand on a step or box **(A)**, then step your left leg onto the floor behind you; bend both knees to lower until your right knee is bent at least 90 degrees **(B)**. Push through the right heel to return to the start. That's 1 rep. Repeat on the other leg and continue alternating for 40 seconds. Rest 20 seconds, then continue to the next exercise.

2

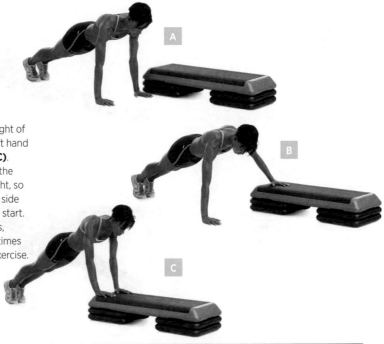

PRESS-UP PLANK WALKOVER

Start in a press-up position to the right of a low box or step **(A)**. Place your left hand onto the step **(B)**, then your right **(C)**. Place your left hand on the floor to the left of the step, followed by your right, so that both hands are now on the left side of the step. Reverse to return to the start. That's 1 rep. Continue for 10 seconds, then rest 10 seconds. Repeat three times (1 minute), then move to the next exercise.

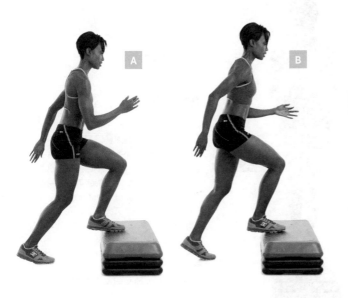

3

SCISSOR SWITCHES

Place the ball of your left foot on the step in front of you **(A)**. Press onto the box and jump, switching feet so that your right foot is on the step **(B)**. That's 1 rep. Continue alternating as quickly as possible for 10 seconds, then rest 10 seconds. Repeat three times (1 minute). Rest 20 seconds, then move on to the next exercise.

4

PLANK WITH ALTERNATING LEG RAISE

Place your forearms on the step, elbows directly under your shoulders and extend your feet behind you **(A)**. Keeping your core tight and your back flat, raise your right leg off the ground **(B)**. Hold for 3 seconds, then lower and repeat with the other leg. Continue alternating for 30 seconds. Rest 30 seconds, then move to the next exercise.

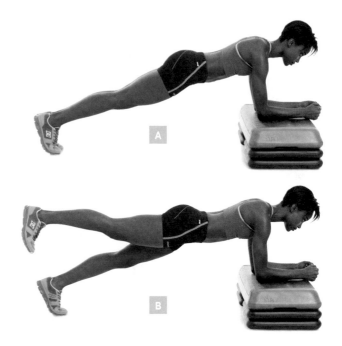

5

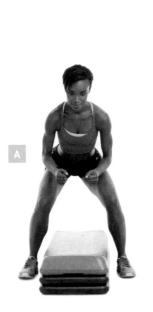

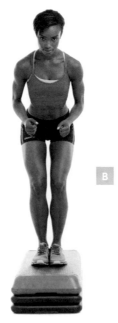

SQUAT AND POP

Place one foot on either side of the step (the narrow portion between your feet); sit your hips back to lower into a half squat, keeping your chest up **(A)**. Quickly jump both feet up onto the box **(B)**, landing softly and immediately jumping to the start, lowering into another squat. That's 1 rep. Continue for 30 seconds, then continue immediately to the next exercise.

6

SIDE PLANK

Place your left forearm on the step directly under your shoulder; extend your legs and raise your hips so that your body forms a straight line from head to heels. Hold for 20 seconds, then immediately switch sides and repeat. Rest 20 seconds, then continue to the next exercise.

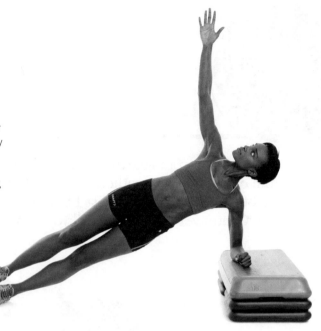

7

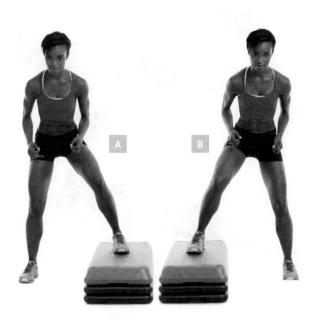

THE RUNAROUND

Stand to the side of the step, knees and elbows slightly bent. Quickly step your left foot onto the step **(A)**, followed by your right, and then quickly step off to the other side, your left foot **(B)** followed by your right. Reverse the movement to return to the starting position. Repeat the lateral step over, then run forward and make a circle around the entire step. That's 1 rep. Immediately repeat the lateral step overs, and continue this pattern for 40 seconds. Rest 40 seconds, then repeat the circuit one more time.

Circuit 1
THE BALL THAT DOES IT ALL

Starting with Circuit 1, complete the prescribed number of reps for each exercise, moving from one to the next without resting. Rest up to a minute, then repeat twice, for a total of three circuits. Rest 1 to 2 minutes, then continue to Circuit 2 and repeat. Continue this pattern until you've finished the workout.

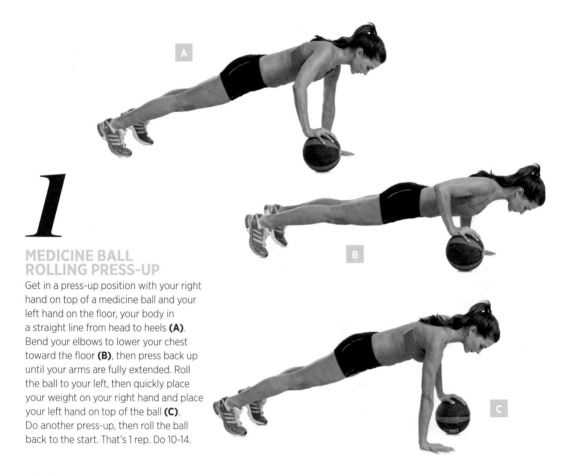

1

MEDICINE BALL ROLLING PRESS-UP

Get in a press-up position with your right hand on top of a medicine ball and your left hand on the floor, your body in a straight line from head to heels **(A)**. Bend your elbows to lower your chest toward the floor **(B)**, then press back up until your arms are fully extended. Roll the ball to your left, then quickly place your weight on your right hand and place your left hand on top of the ball **(C)**. Do another press-up, then roll the ball back to the start. That's 1 rep. Do 10-14.

2

MEDICINE BALL HIP RAISE

Lie face up on the floor, arms out to your sides with palms up, and place both feet on a medicine ball, knees bent about 90 degrees **(A)**. Squeeze your glutes and raise your hips so that your body forms a straight line from shoulders to knees **(B)**. Pause, then lower back to the start. That's 1 rep. Do 15.

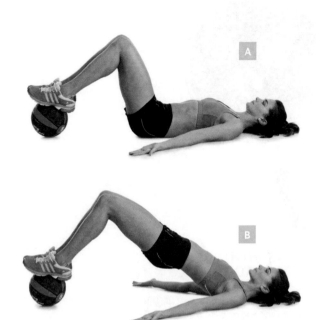

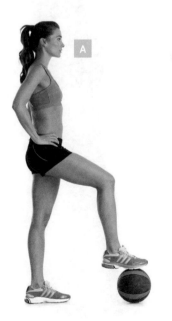

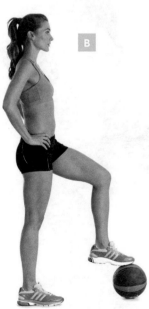

3

MEDICINE BALL TAPS

Place a medicine ball on the ground in front of you and lightly place one foot on top of it, knee bent **(A)**. Keeping your weight over your hips, switch feet so the other foot is on top of the ball **(B)**; continue alternating as quickly as possible, picking your knees up and staying light on the balls of your feet. Do as many taps as you can in 1 minute.

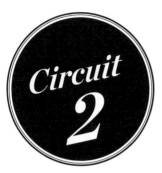

1

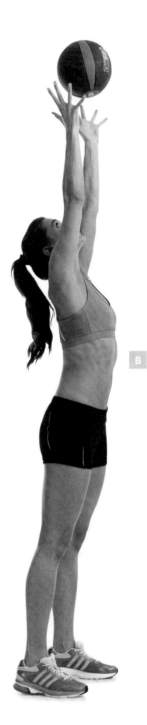

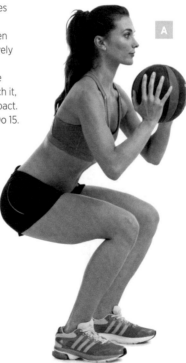

SQUAT WITH OVERHEAD TOSS

Stand with your feet hip-width apart holding a medicine ball at chest height, elbows bent and close to the body. Sit your hips back and bend your knees to lower your body until your thighs are parallel to the floor **(A)**. Pause, then press through your heels and explosively return to standing as you straighten your arms to press the ball toward the ceiling, releasing it overhead **(B)**. Catch it, bending your knees to absorb the impact. Immediately lower into another rep. Do 15.

A

B

2

MEDICINE BALL DONKEY KICKS

Place the medicine ball on the floor and extend your legs behind you into a press-up position, feet wider than hip-width apart and hands on top of the ball. Keeping your core tight, bend your right knee toward your chest **(A)**, pause, then press your heel up toward the ceiling, knee bent at 90 degrees **(B)**. That's 1 rep. Immediately draw the knee back into the chest and continue for 10 reps, then switch sides and repeat.

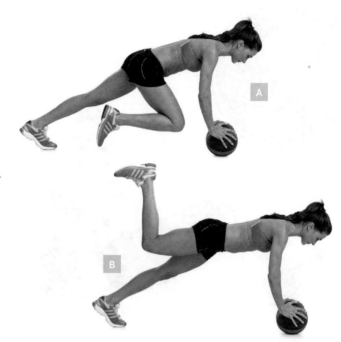

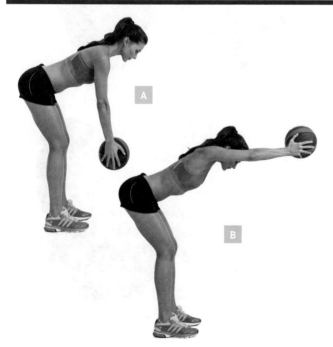

3

Bent-Over Arm Raise

Holding a medicine ball with both hands, stand with your feet about shoulder-width apart, knees slightly bent. Hinge forward at the hips to lower your torso toward the floor, keeping your back flat, arms hanging straight in line with your shoulders **(A)**. Keeping your arms straight and without changing the position of your torso, brace your core and raise the ball until your arms are on either side of your head **(B)**. Pause, then slowly lower back to the start. That's 1 rep. Do 12-15.

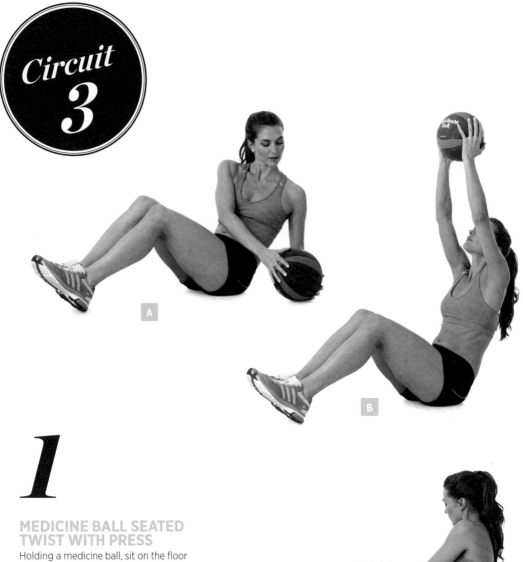

Circuit 3

1

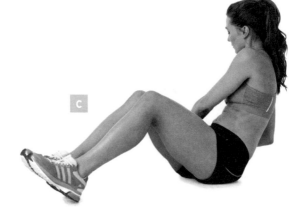

MEDICINE BALL SEATED TWIST WITH PRESS

Holding a medicine ball, sit on the floor with your knees bent and feet flexed. Keep your back straight and hips facing forward as you twist your torso to the left and touch the weight to the floor next to you **(A)**. Rotate back to the centre and press the ball overhead **(B)**, then lower it and rotate to the left **(C)**. Reverse the movement to return to the start. That's 1 rep. Do 10.

2

MEDICINE BALL BURPEE

Stand with your feet slightly wider than shoulder-width apart, holding a medicine ball at your chest **(A)**. Push your hips back, bend your knees, and squat down to place the ball on the floor with both hands on the ball **(B)**. Kick your legs back into a press-up position **(C)**; quickly reverse the movement to return to standing. That's 1 rep. Do 15.

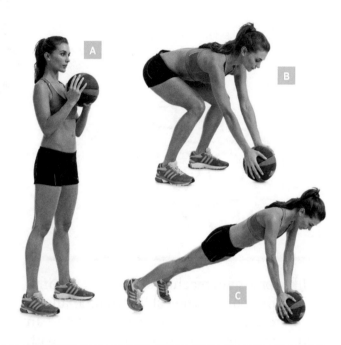

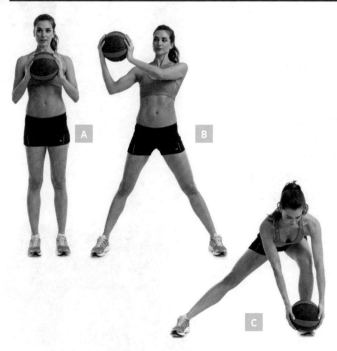

3

AROUND-THE -WORLD LUNGE

Hold a medicine ball in front of your chest, feet shoulder-width apart **(A)**. Take a big step to your left, lowering your body by pushing your hips back and bending your left knee as you circle the ball to the right **(B)** and bring it over your left foot **(C)**. Press through your left heel to return to the start. That's 1 rep. Repeat on the other side, and continue alternating for a total of 20 reps.

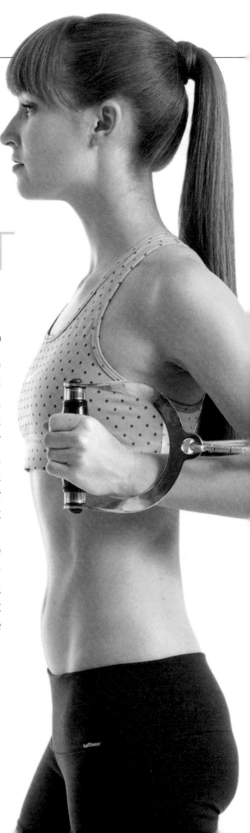

SCULPT A KNOCKOUT BODY

Unlike some gym machines, that lock you into a fixed movement, the cable machine allows for more functional movements, so you can work your muscles from all angles with a greater range of motion. It also keeps your muscles under constant tension, giving you a tough workout, especially your core, which has to work overtime to stabilise your body. You can get a killer head-to-toe workout without hopping around the gym.

This routine is designed to build lean muscle and up your calorie burn during – and after – the workout. Complete 12-15 reps of each exercise, moving from one to the next without a break. Rest for 1 minute, then repeat the circuit three times.

1

CABLE SQUAT TO ROW

Grab a universal grip (a strap with two handles) in each hand and stand facing the weight stack, feet hip-width apart. Sit your hips back and bend your knees to lower your body toward the floor **(A)**. As you stand, bend your elbows to row the handles to the sides of your chest **(B)**. That's 1 rep.

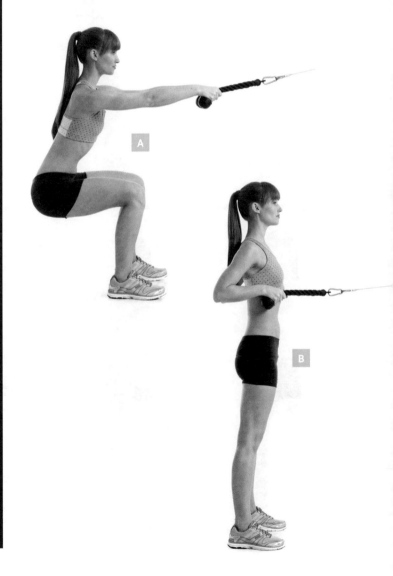

4

SINGLE-ARM CABLE CHEST PRESS

Grab a handle (attached at chest height) with your left hand and face away from the machine, elbow bent and palm down. Step your left foot back into a split stance, knees bent **(A)**. Brace your abs and forcefully press the handle forward **(B)**. Do all reps, then switch sides and repeat.

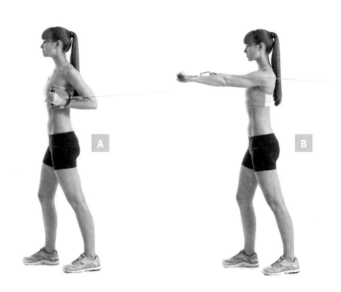

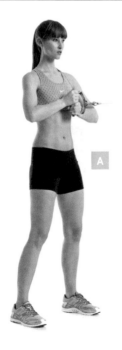
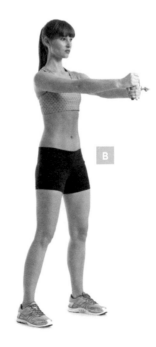

5

CABLE CORE PRESS

Stand to the right of the cable station and grab the handle (attached at chest height) with both hands at your chest **(A)**. Keeping a tight core, press the handle directly out in front of you **(B)**. Hold for 2 seconds, then return to start. Complete all reps on that side, then turn to face the opposite direction and repeat.

6

CABLE WOODCHOPPER

Secure a handle at the highest point and stand to the right of the machine. Grab the handle with both hands so your arms are extended above your left shoulder, feet wide and knees slightly bent **(A)**. Keeping your arms straight, pull the handle across the front of your body to the outside of your right thigh, shifting your weight from your left foot to your right **(B)**. Slowly return to start. That's 1 rep. Do all reps on that side, then switch sides and repeat.

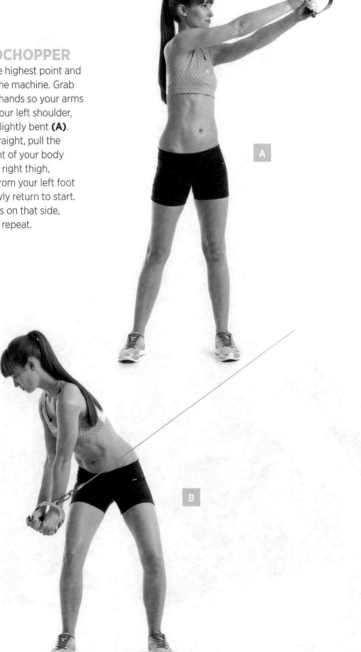

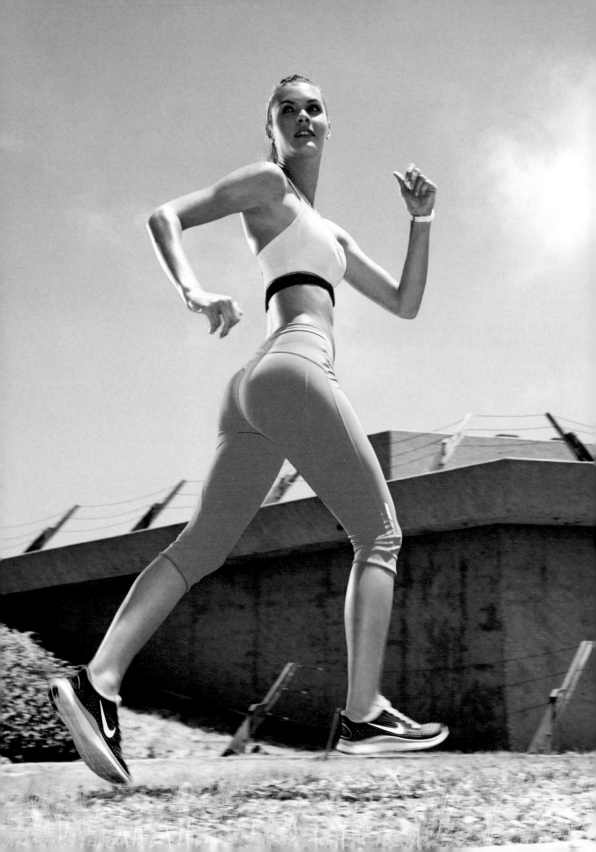

CRUSH
MORE
CALORIES

Rethink your cardio routine for better results in less time

These quick-but-killer efforts may be the closest thing you'll find to a magic calorie-burning bullet. You'll spend less time working out, but continue to incinerate calories at an increased rate, even during your recovery periods. This kind of training builds muscle, prevents plateaus and increases endurance. It also busts boredom, boosts confidence and improves mental toughness, giving you strength to keep going when your body wants to stop. But use these sessions sparingly. Slip just one of these workouts into your weekly routine. And don't just stick with the one that feels easiest: mix and match to keep your body guessing.

7 FAT-BLASTING CARDIO WORKOUTS

Comfort zone, be damned. Add these plateau busters to your regime to keep your body guessing

The mile challenge

Runners, whether you want to set a new personal best at your next race or just want a workout that tests and improves your maximum speed, try this:

A Break down the total distance into smaller increments and calculate the speed required at each in order to complete the entire distance at your desired pace. So if you want to run a 6-minute mile, you have to be able to run:

- A half-mile in 3 minutes
- A quarter-mile in 90 seconds
- 200 metres in 45 seconds
- 100 metres in 22.5 seconds

B Run a repeat at the longest distance you can make the time. (Can't make the 100-metre time? Readjust your per-mile pace.)

C Rest three times as long as the length of the interval (so for 200 metres, that's 2 minutes and 15 seconds).

D Continue the repeats until you can no longer maintain 90% of the speed. (Figure it out by dividing the time by 0.9. So 200-metre repeats are continued until you can no longer make it in 50 seconds.)

Cardio climber

Try this 'ladder' interval drill, climbing up (run gradually longer intervals) or down (run gradually shorter intervals). Run 1 minute hard, 2 minutes easy, 2 minutes hard, 3 minutes easy, 3 minutes hard, 4 minutes easy, and then work back down.

Flip on your fat-burners

Some interval workouts are are just too complicated. This one couldn't be any easier – to remember, that is. Researchers found that people who followed a programme similar to this 3 times a week for 2 weeks saw the same benefits as those who completed 10 hours of moderate exercise during the 2 weeks. So you'll improve your body's efficiency in one-fifth of the time. After a short warm up, complete the following workout, repeating the pattern 10 times. Finish with a 3-to-5-minute cooldown.

ON: SPRINT!	OFF: RECOVER!
For 1 minute, run at a pace that leaves you winded, but not breathless. (Think 8/10, with 10 being your top speed.)	For 1 minute, jog or walk. (You should be able to speak comfortably by the end.)

Calorie-shredding shuttle

This simple cardio drill will raise your heart rate and incinerate calories. Find 30 feet of open space and place three markers in a line, 15 feet apart. Straddling the middle marker, sprint to your right and touch the line with your right hand. Turn and sprint back to your left for 30 feet and touch with your left hand; turn once more and sprint back to your starting point. That's 1 rep (it should take 5-7 seconds). Rest for 25 seconds, and on your next rep, move to your left first. Continue this pattern until you've completed 10 reps.

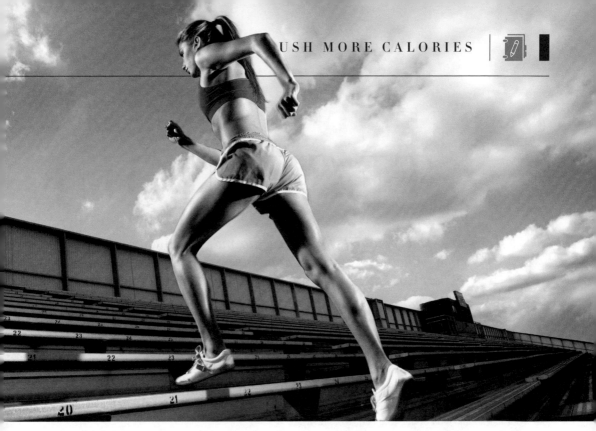

20-minute tempo runs

0-5 mins	Warm up (easy effort; you can sing at this pace)
5-7 mins	Moderate effort (you can carry on a conversation)
7-10 mins	Hard effort (you can speak only a few words at a time)
10-12 mins	Moderate effort
12-14 mins	Recovery (easy effort)
14-16 mins	Very hard effort (you're huffing and puffing too much to talk)
16-20 mins	Cooldown (easy effort)

Build-up basics

Use this template for a tempo plan that revs up your metabolism anytime, anywhere.

2 mins	Easy-moderate (4/10 intensity level)	
2 mins	Moderate (5/10 intensity)	**x3**
1 min	Hard (8/10 intensity)	
+ 5 mins	Easy (3/10 intensity)	

1-minute speed intervals

Many speed workouts come with two training speeds: superfast or barely moving. This plan adds a third, moderate speed into each 1-minute interval segment. This tweak helps exercisers maintain a higher heart rate for longer, which builds endurance and speed faster. A study published in the *Journal of Applied Physiology* reported that exercisers who followed this routine for 20-30 minutes were able to drop a minute off their 5K times. Warm up, follow this 30-20-10-second plan, then finish with a short cooldown.

0:00-0:30	Jog at a slow pace
0:31-0:50	Run at a moderate pace
0:51-1:00	Sprint
1:01-5:00	Repeat the 30-20-10 interval (five times total)
5:01-6:59	Walk
7:00-7:30	Jog at a slow pace
7:31-7:50	Run at a moderate pace
7:51-8:00	Sprint
8:01-12:00	Repeat the 30-20-10 interval (five times total)

PERFECT YOUR
TECHNIQUE

Whatever your favourite form of cardio, make sure you're doing it right. Whether it's running, cycling or swimming, these expert tips will help you do it better and avoid injury

A runner's guide

Running isn't a requirement for fat loss but it can be your most accessible tool. All you need is your sports bra and trainers.

Fast feet. Take quick, short steps instead of longer strides, which can hurt your lower back and tire you out. Your feet should land under your centre of gravity, not out in front of you.

Soft steps. Land lightly between your heel and midfoot, and let your foot roll smoothly forward. Push off with your toes.

Head up. Look ahead and scan the horizon to prevent slouching (unless you're running on a trail or other bumpy surface).

Straight swing. Relax your arms and bend them about 90 degrees, letting them swing front to back (not across your midline) between waist and lower-chest level. Keep your hands loose – think about lightly holding a piece of paper between your thumb and index finger.

Lean in. Lean forward from your hips to maintain momentum without sacrificing your posture. (To get the approximate feel, stand still on both feet, then shift your weight toward the balls of your feet without lifting your heels.)

Proud chest. Keep your chest lifted, shoulders stretching down your back. Imagine there is a string attached to your sternum pulling you upward as you run.

A swimmer's guide

Front crawl is a perfect stroke for calorie burn and muscle recruitment. Each stroke is like a mini resistance workout for your entire body.

Keep your head down. Align your head and neck with your spine, and keep your shoulders relaxed. Look at the black line on the bottom of the pool with your head in a neutral position. This will prevent your hips from sinking and keep your body level in the water.

Roll over. As you rotate your body to the side to breathe, rotate your head (don't lift it out of the water) and take a breath through your mouth. Exhale gently and gradually under the water until your next breath.

Do arm circles. Pull through the water, keeping your fingers pointed toward the bottom of the pool. Your hand should trace an imaginary line on the pool's bottom. Finish each stroke by extending your arm fully behind you until your hand is close to your thigh.

Open your hands. Avoid cupping your hands. When they're relaxed, with your fingers slightly open, they'll propel you forward more easily.

Keep your elbows up. Your elbows should always be higher than your wrist.

Use your hips. The kick starts in the hips and core. Imagine you're trying to kick off a pair of flip-flops in the water.

Kick it with fast feet. Keep your feet close together and in line with the rest of your body. They should be pointed naturally, fluttering at about six kicks per stroke.

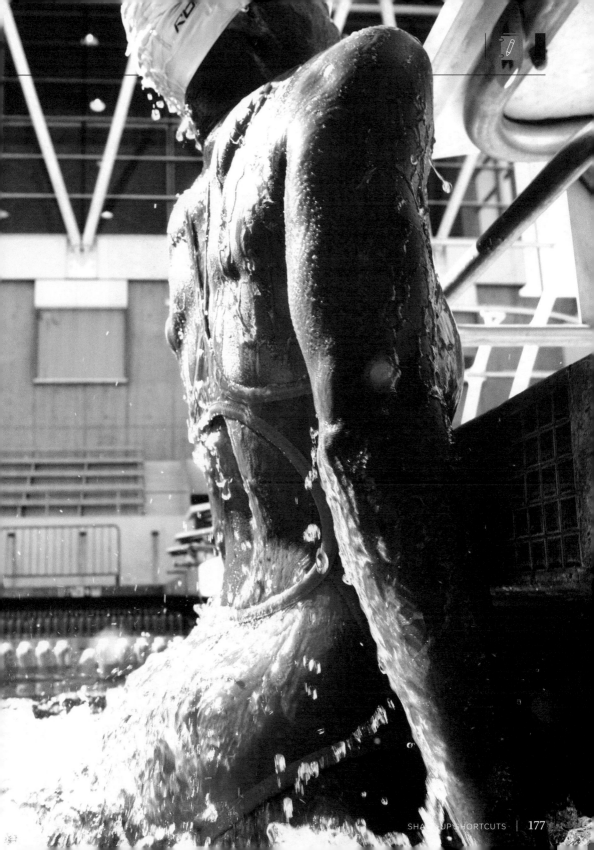

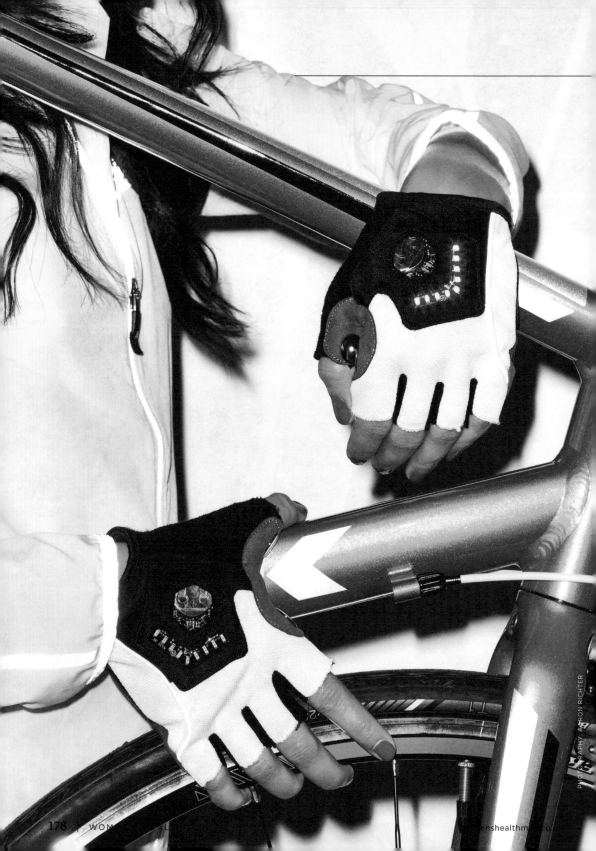

A cyclist's guide

Whether you're sweating away in spin class or out on the open road, there's a better way to ride your bike.

Pedal smoothly. Cycle in fluid circles rather than jamming down on the pedals. To do this, push down on the pedal with the ball of your foot; next, pull your foot through the bottom of the stroke, then pull up and back around – cleat pedals, where you 'click in' with cycling shoes, are a big help here. Aim for about 90 rpm (to calculate rpm, count how many times your right knee comes up in 60 seconds).

Eyes on the prize. Resist the urge to put your head down when you're going hard or getting tired. It can slow your oxygen intake, tiring you out faster. (Plus, you're much more likely to crash.)

Core performance. While your legs are busy pumping, keep your upper body still – don't rock side to side, especially while climbing. Maintain an aerodynamically flat back and keep your elbows bent and relaxed (it helps absorb shock when you hit a bump outside). Hold your arms in line with your body, not out to the side. Keeping your upper body relaxed will reduce strain on your lower back.

Take a seat. Your weight should feel evenly distributed, with 60% on the saddle (seat) and 40% on the handlebar. The saddle height should be positioned so there's a slight bend in your knee when your foot is at the bottom of a stroke. Most of all, you should be comfortable. Your best bet? Get a professional bike fit at a shop. It will cost upwards of £100 but it's worth it.

Get up. Sitting is the most efficient way to ride – you can use up to 10% more energy when you're out of the saddle. But sometimes, for instance when you're climbing a monster hill, you need extra power. When you stand, all of your body weight pushes down on the pedals, giving each stroke more oomph. If you stand, shift into a harder gear so your legs don't circle too quickly. Rise up, and keep your bum over the seat.

BIKE YOUR WAY TO A BETTER BODY

Cycling is a multitasking cardio workout that fries fat and demolishes stress without pounding your body into the ground. Here's how it can make you a lean, fat-burning machine

It torches calories. Even pedaling at an easy pace, a 130-pound woman will torch 473 calories in an hour. Upping the speed to 14 to 16 mph burns close to 591 calories.

It sculpts killer legs. Your quads, glutes, and calves are keeping you moving. To better engage these muscles, focus on your pedal stroke. Try to make a perfect circle: Push forward and then down with your quads; pull back with your hamstrings, as if you're wiping mud off the bottom of your shoe; and then use your calves and hip flexors to pull up and back.

It saves your joints. Riding a bike puts a lot less stress on the knees, ankles, and spine than walking or running. You can develop muscle power and cardio endurance without feeling the same impact.

It tones all over. Pedaling while standing engages your core and triceps as you stabilise your body over the bike. Spend roughly half the time pedaling out of the saddle, focusing on keeping your core tight.

It protects your ticker. Heart disease is the second-largest killer of UK women, and two top risk factors are high blood pressure and LDL cholesterol. In one study, researchers asked 32 women to cycle for 30 minutes, three times a week. After a year, they'd lowered their blood pressure and LDL, and increased their aerobic fitness.

WORK OUT
THE KINKS

Tend to aching muscles with this foam-roller routine. The moves take about 10 to 15 minutes to complete, and hit all the places where you're most prone to soreness. Plus, you can do them anytime – during your favourite TV show, before bed, first thing in the morning or after a workout. Roll over each spot five to 10 times. If a spot feels way too tender, try starting below the area, work up to it and hold for a few seconds, then roll through it.

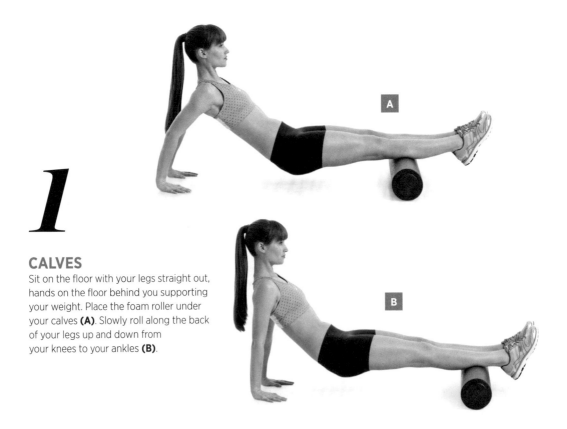

1

CALVES

Sit on the floor with your legs straight out, hands on the floor behind you supporting your weight. Place the foam roller under your calves **(A)**. Slowly roll along the back of your legs up and down from your knees to your ankles **(B)**.

2

HAMSTRINGS

Sit with your right leg on the roller; bend your left knee, cross your left ankle over your right ankle, and put your hands on the floor behind you **(A)**. Roll up and down from your knee to just under your right bum cheek **(B)**. Switch legs.

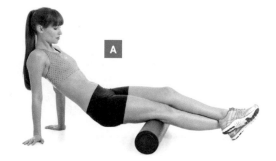

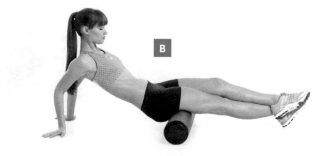

3

QUADS

Lie face down on the floor and place the roller under your hips **(A)**. Lean on your left leg **(B)** and roll up and down from your hip to your knee. Switch legs.

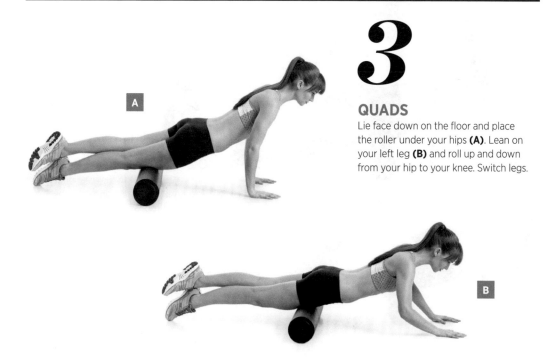

4

BACK

Sit on the floor with the foam roller on your lower back, resting your hands behind you for balance **(A)**. Tighten your abs and slowly bend your knees to move the roller up your back, just below your shoulder blades **(B)**.

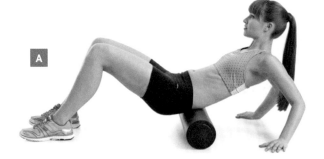

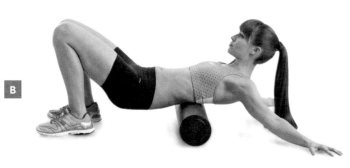

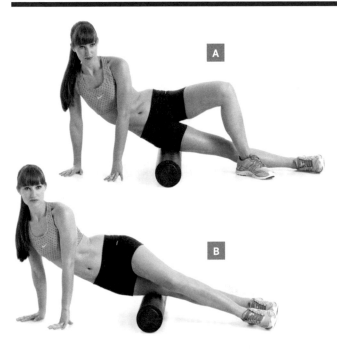

5

OUTER THIGHS

Lie on your side with the roller under your right hip **(A)**. Bracing your abs and glutes for balance, slowly roll down from your hip to your knee **(B)**. Switch to the other side and repeat.

6

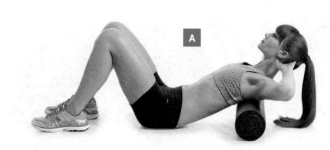

SHOULDERS AND SIDES

Lie on your back with the roller behind your shoulders. Lace your fingers loosely behind your head and lean your upper back into the roller **(A)**. Brace your abs and glutes for stability, and slowly press into the roller on your left side, raising your right shoulder **(B)**. Roll from your underarms to the bottom of your rib cage. Return to the centre and switch sides.

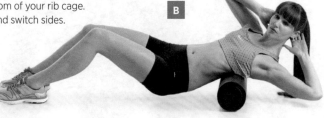

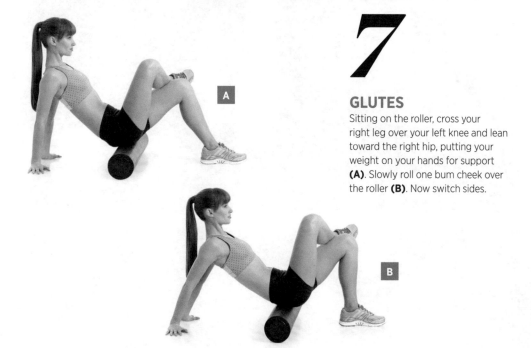

7

GLUTES

Sitting on the roller, cross your right leg over your left knee and lean toward the right hip, putting your weight on your hands for support **(A)**. Slowly roll one bum cheek over the roller **(B)**. Now switch sides.

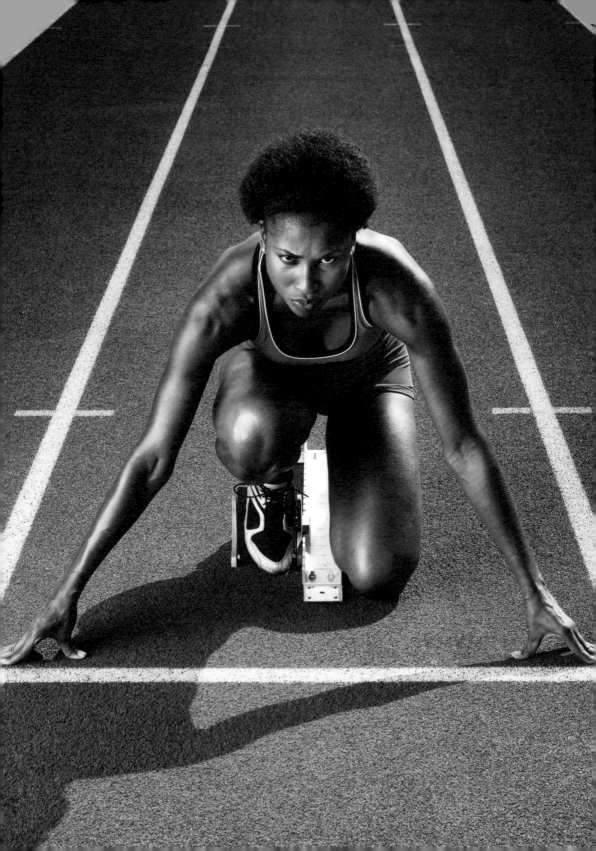

STAYING
ON
TRACK

How to keep your fitness focus when real life gets in the way

···

You've made a great start to your fitness regime, you're seeing results and, despite the hard, hard work you're enjoying it and anticipating further progress. You deserve to be pleased with yourself – but be careful. Motivation can waver as the your body learns to compensate for your increased effort. Or you can find yourself becoming bored at the prospect of yet more burpees. But there are ways to banish these bugbears before they lead to burnout. We'll show you how maintain your focus by varying your workout, enlisting friends and colleagues and finding new inspiration in your exercises. Onwards and upwards, always.

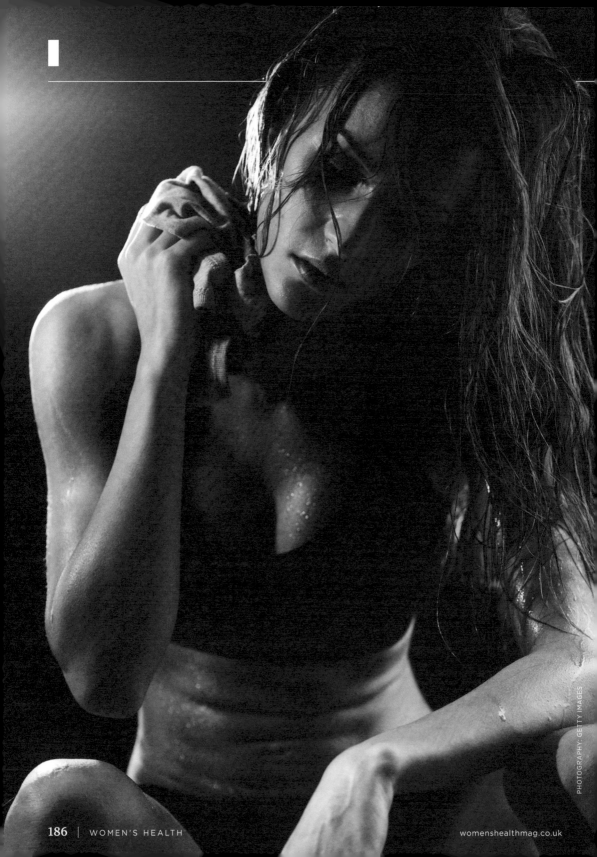

THE
FOUR STAGES
OF
EXERCISE BURNOUT

Watch out for the warning signs, to avoid an exercise slump

STAGE 1 The honeymoon

You're determined to look hot at your best friend's wedding, so you ramp up your workouts to six or seven days a week – and you never miss a single session. **STAY ON TRACK** Take a less-is-more approach. Burnout often happens when you expect too much too soon. Even with the smartest, most effective workout regime, you still can't force your body to become stronger or slimmer any faster than it can physiologically manage. Don't exceed your ability to recover. Start with the lowest reps, sets, and weights. Gradually increase exercise volume and intensity to avoid injury – and always schedule at least one full day off. Recovery days are essential.

STAGE 2 Disenchantment

Your excitement fades when you don't see results right away. You stop looking forward to gym time and start slacking during – or just plain skipping – workouts. **STAY ON TRACK** According to research, simply having a supportive friend, family member, or significant other makes you more likely to stick with your fitness regimen. Participants who started a new workout plan with a partner cheering them on logged more exercise hours than people who lacked this support.

STAGE 3 Stalling

Boredom and apathy override your commitment and motivation. You'll use almost anything – work, family, stress, the weather – as an excuse to skip exercise. **STAY ON TRACK** Once women work hard to master a new skill, they stick with it because, hey, they can do it. But it also impedes progress and breeds boredom. Instead of fixating on a far-off finish line (like losing a certain number of pounds), shift your attention to the instant rewards you can reap – like feeling happier and more energetic.

STAGE 4 Frustration and surrender

Exercise slides from your list of top priorities. All you want to do is throw in the towel. **STAY ON TRACK** Register for a race that requires you to raise sponsorship. You're far less likely to bail if you've asked your friends and colleagues to donate. Still not working? Put money on the line. Experts say people will work twice as hard when money is at stake, compared with relying only on willpower. Make a friendly wager among colleagues and friends. Everyone puts £20 in the kitty and whoever scores the most workout sessions over three months wins the pot.

OUTSMART FITNESS
ROADBLOCKS

Maybe you've fallen in love! Or perhaps you're working too hard. Whatever the distraction, these strategies will keep you on track for a hotter, healthier body

You work insane hours

You're putting in 12-hour work days that don't leave much time for runs in the park.

TRAINING TIP Plan workouts when you have the fewest conflicts, which for most people is first thing. Not an early riser? Inch your alarm back a little every few days; it will gradually reset your body-clock, and eventually, you'll be waking up half an hour earlier, no problem – giving plenty of time to fit in any workout from Reshape Your Body on page 89. If you prefer to hit the gym at night, get changed before you leave work. Otherwise, it can be tempting to head straight home.

MENTAL TRICK Not only can daily exercise help your mental sharpness, learning, and memory, it'll boost your work productivity. A recent study found that women working out three or more times a week earn 10% more, thanks to the extra energy it brings.

You're in the new-love bubble

Morning exercisers find it tough to get out of bed when there's someone new and irresistible lying next to them – and sex makes for great exercise, doesn't it? Whereas, evening exercisers often have a hard time passing up romantic dinners in favour of the gym.

TRAINING TIP Work out when they're not around – either during your lunch break or as part of a girls' night (meet up for a spin class and then head to dinner). Or, get your lover to do it with you. Working out together can improve communication, strengthen mutual support, and give you more shared interests.

MENTAL TRICK Exercise can do more to boost your sex life than sharing a bottle of wine. Research shows that frequent exercisers feel more sexually desirable. And, yes, spending time together is important, but one study found that women who do their own thing have happier marriages. So it'll suit both parties if 'me time' spent in the gym makes you feel sexier.

You were sidelined by injury

People either rush into their previous workouts, which puts them at risk of another injury, or are so afraid of getting hurt again that they put it off altogether.

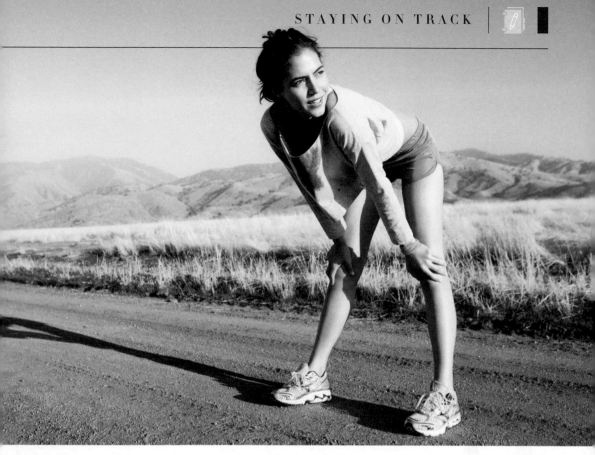

TRAINING TIP After your doctor clears you, scale back your old routine by at least 50% for the first two weeks or so. Back off a bit whenever the area feels tender or painful, or you could ultimately throw off your form and develop new injuries.

MENTAL TRICK Challenge those negative, 'poor me' thoughts. Staying positive may sound like psychobabble, but it really works. And while it's normal to be nervous, it's important to trust your doctor's advice and start gently when he gives you the go-ahead.

Your social calendar has cramped your gym time

Weeks of eating, drinking and partying (and not exercising) have left you feeling overwhelmed by the idea of having to undo the damage.

TRAINING TIP Hitting the gym hard can quickly lead to burnout. Rather than doubling your sessions or hours of cardio, start by keeping it manageable, with yoga or short strength circuits.

MENTAL TRICK Don't give in to 'It's too late now'

thinking. Remember that it's easier to drop 2lbs now than wait until you need to lose 10. You don't have to give up all indulgences immediately. Make one healthy swap or change each day to ease you back on track.

Of course you're exhausted, you've just had a baby

Intense exercise is usually off-limits for six weeks postpartum. After that, sheer exhaustion can keep new mums on the sofa.

TRAINING TIP Even if you're wiped, pop in a DVD or slip your baby in the stroller for a brisk walk. It will boost your energy and help you sleep better. And exercising helps fend off postnatal depression.

MENTAL TRICK Women can get obsessed with dropping the baby weight and get frustrated if it doesn't happen right away. But that just adds stress. Make your goal more realistic and you'll be more likely to tackle it. Mentally commit to just 5 -10 minutes of exercise. If you don't feel energised once you get to the end of it, try again later, or take the day off and try again tomorrow.

STAY
MOTIVATED

*Focus on the immediate pay offs,
so exercise becomes your priority*

Researchers recently reported that women who tracked instant results after a workout – like feeling happier and more energetic – exercised 34% more over a year than those who focused on weight-loss or appearance goals. It makes sense. Physical changes can take months, and tasks that don't have tangible, immediate payoffs can fall off your checklist. Start noticing how you feel after your workouts. Are you more self-confident? Less stressed? Find the payoffs that are most important to you: it will ensure that you prioritise exercise in your routine.

Get ahead at work

Aiming for a promotion? Don't sacrifice gym time for late nights at work. Researchers found that women who exercise at least twice a week feel more in control of their jobs and find them less demanding than those who don't work out. According to a survey in the *International Journal of Workplace Health Management*, workers who exercised reported a 32% increase in motivation and a 28% increase in time management compared to the days they didn't work out.

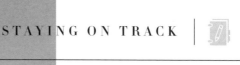
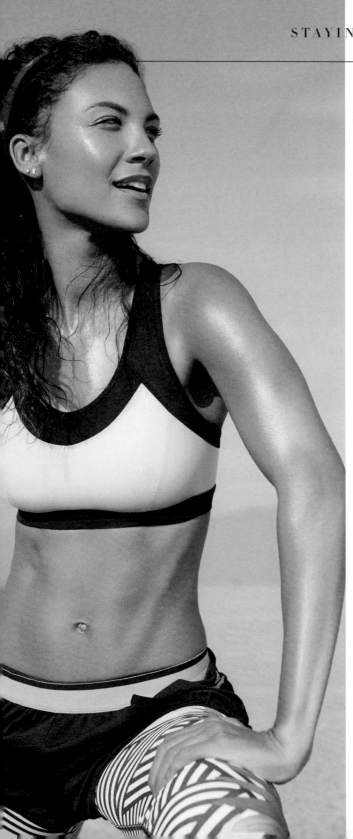

Think sharper

According to a study published in *Clinical Neurophysiology*, 20 minutes of moderate exercise immediately increases attention and cognitive ability. There's a shift in brain activity that enhances executive functioning, which plans, schedules, and coordinates thoughts and actions. This amplified focus can last up to an hour, so schedule a quick workout before a time when you'll really need to be on form.

Get glowing skin

As your heart rate rises, the increase in blood flow circulates to the surface of your skin, giving you that revitalising flush of colour. Sweating is good for your skin, too. Some of the water evaporates to cool the body, and the rest is reabsorbed into the skin, giving it a nicely hydrated look post-workout.

Have hotter sex

A study published in the *Journal of Sexual Medicine* found that women who completed a 20-minute treadmill run before watching an erotic film clocked a 150% increase in arousal. It might be best to exercise at home – the uptick in arousal lasts about 30 minutes.

Sleep better

Working out zaps stress and anxiety, and helps your body regulate its own temperature – all of which means more restful sleep. According to a study published in the US journal *Mental Health and Physical Activity*, participants who engaged in moderately intense exercise for 150 minutes a week fell asleep faster and felt less tired during the day. It doesn't matter what time of day you choose to workout, either. Only limited research suggests that late-night physical activity affects your sleep.

INDEX

Women'sHealth

Editor **Shoshana Goldberg**
Art Director **Graeme Sapsed**
Sub Editor **Charlie Jackson**
Picture Editor **Celia Topping**
Production **Roger Bilsland**

Group Publishing Director **Alun Williams**　　Ad Manager **Chloe Barrington**
Sales Director **Luke Robins**　　Marketing Director **Claire Matthews**

CEO, HEARST MAGAZINES UK
Anna Jones

HEARST-RODALE JOINT BOARD OF DIRECTORS
President and CEO, Hearst Magazines International
Duncan Edwards
Finance Director, Hearst Magazines UK **Claire Blunt**
Senior Vice President, Rodale International
Robert Novick

HEARST MAGAZINES UK
Director of Circulation **Reid Holland**
HR Director **Surinder Simmons**
Head of Newstrade Marketing **Jennifer Smith**
Circulation Manager **Bianca Lloyd-King**

RODALE INTERNATIONAL
**Rodale Inc, 33 East Minor Street,
Emmaus, Pennsylvania 18098, USA**

Editorial Director, Rodale International **John Ville**
Editorial Director Women's Health **Laura Ongaro**
Deputy Editorial Director **Veronika Taylor**
International Content Manager **Karl Rozemeyer**
Editorial Assistant **Natanya Spies**
Director Business Development **Kevin LaBonge**
International Business Manager **Seana Williams**
Business Coordinator **Hannah Roshetko**

Hearst-Rodale Ltd, 33 Broadwick Street, London, W1F 0DQ Tel: 020 7339 4400 Fax: 020 7339 4420

Workout photography: Beth Bischoff